BLUE MOON VEGETARIAN
REFLECTIONS, RECIPES, AND ADVICE FOR A PLANT-BASED DIET

BY PAULA MARIE COOMER

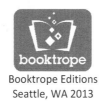

booktrope

Booktrope Editions
Seattle, WA 2013

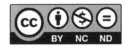
Editor: Julie Molinari

Cover Designer: Kelsey Grafton

PRINT ISBN: 978-1-62015-137-2

EPUB ISBN: 978-1-62015-082-5

Library of Congress Control Number: 2013919886

For Katie and Suzi

"Once the realization is accepted that even between the closest human beings infinite distances continue, a wonderful living side by side can grow, if they succeed in loving the distance between them which makes it possible for each to see the other whole against the sky."

—RANIER MARIA RILKE

"A man of my spiritual intensity does not eat corpses."

—George Bernard Shaw

FULL MOON

NINETEEN YEARS. Nineteen years since a blue moon coincided with New Year's Eve the way it did at the feeble end of 2009. A year to make me say thank goodness when it was finally gone. Just a day before I'd learned of the death of beloved experimental writer Raymond Federmann, with whom I'd studied when he came to the University of Idaho as a distinguished visiting writer back in the 1990s. A professor who spent a week sewing feathers onto our wings, daring us to chart our own routes, and who relished riding around in our grungy cars and hanging with us during the after-hours. The fifth of my life's top influential people to leave the planet in 2009.

The year was enough to awaken the curmudgeon in me: first, a long-awaited vacation in San Francisco, my favorite city and a place to which I'd waited thirty years to return, botched by a torn meniscus.

Then, knee surgery and months of leaning-on-a-cane recovery, during which my father's heart had to be opened and reorganized. My best friend/father Frankensteinerized, zippered in the chest.

And his daughter the nurse, incapacitated herself, two thousand miles away.

A year of chaos.

What's worse is that I'd allowed those losses to overshadow the good things about 2009: my youngest son's wedding to a woman we all adored; several trips prior to the San Francisco trip—some for work and some with my fiancé, my engagement to whom also occurred in 2009 after nearly twenty years of singledom—to Oregon, Illinois, Massachusetts, Kentucky, and Texas; as well as a novel I wrote recorded for radio and having a go as an audiobook.

The last blue moon on New Year's Eve occurred in 1990, which was the year my second marriage fell apart, the year I began weightlifting, and the year I became a vegetarian for the first time. I say first because I was about to do it again, coinciding with this New Year's Eve blue moon. Beginning January 1, 2010, my status as your average organic-foods omnivore would expire. A little dairy, still, perhaps, in the form of yogurt and half 'n' half, since it would take the planet slipping off-course to unbind me from coffee, a thing I've repeatedly declared I endure only as an accompaniment to cream. Once in a while, eggs. But no more animal flesh. No more creatures of the sea. I was doing it because, having turned fifty-three in September, and having been told by my medical practitioner, "It's time," to start chewing that daily baby aspirin, and having a father and grandmother who developed Type 2 diabetes at just my stage of life, and having gained more than one hundred pounds since I started eating meat again, stopped weightlifting, and became a writer, I felt I had no recourse. If I wanted to live into the Georgia O'Keefe years—which I did—I was going to have to get fit.

I was also doing it because I'd stopped trusting our food system. Throughout my life I'd eaten almost exclusively organics, and as the daughter of hundreds of years of Scots transplanted to the south-central Kentucky hills and Cherokee and freed Africans, the diets of whom consisted of nothing they did not raise, hunt, or gather themselves, and who knew nothing of fertilizer save manure, and never dreamed of the need for a product such as a pesticide, since they knew which plants repelled such organisms and arranged crops so that one plant protected the next. Laying hens and frying chickens roamed the rows to scavenge rare bugs like tomato cutworms. I had come to suspect my body was genetically programmed only to consume whole foods. In fact, I believed that about us all. My gut had never done well on Doritos and McDonald's, and as the years went on, it wasn't doing so well on muscle fiber.

Whether it was a way of me taking control of my life, or my body sounding its warning bell, I could only say, "Let it begin." It was about seeing what I still had left in me.

My fiancé, Phil, who works as a federal contracting officer, decided to share these goals, sane and pragmatic person that he is. He is also a fabulous cook and an inventor of original dishes. And since 2010 was our wedding year, and we wanted to be healthy and active together for decades more, it made perfect sense that we use the experience of lifestyle change as yet another way to discover the deeper parts of each other.

* * *

New Year's Day brought with it the vegetarian's constant dilemma: how to get enough protein. In fact, it is a joke among vegetarians, since an omnivore's first question upon meeting a vegetarian almost always is, "How do you get your protein?" The problem is not how to get enough protein, but how to get enough *complete* protein. There was a time when some researchers insisted that the only way to get a complete protein—a protein containing all the essential amino acids—was to *eat* a complete protein in the form of fish, eggs, or animal flesh. Others said you could combine incomplete proteins, such as those in grains and legumes, the combined amino acids in each coming together in the gut. Now we understand that as long as all nine amino acids are consumed at some point throughout the day, the body can do what it needs to, and we also know that hemp seed—yes, that lowly little commoner that is cousin to marijuana (and no, you can't get high from consuming it)—contains a complete protein, and pretty much is the only plant source that does.

In fact, hemp seed contains all the essential amino acids and fatty acids. No other single plant source contains these major construction blocks of the human anatomy in such an easily digestible form. Hemp seed is also a strong source for linoleic acid (LA) and linolenic acid (LNA), which are essential fatty acids (EFAs). EFAs govern growth, vitality, and state of mind. LA and LNA are involved in transferring oxygen from the air in the lungs to every cell in the body. They play a part in holding oxygen in the cell membrane where it acts as a barrier to invading viruses and bacteria, neither of which can thrive in the presence of oxygen. The bent shape of the essential fatty acids keeps them from dissolving into each other. They are slippery and will not clog arteries like the sticky straight-shaped saturated fats and the trans-fatty acids in cooking oils and shortenings that are made by super-heating polyunsaturated oils during the refining. (This is why cold-pressed oils are superior and preferable.) LA and LNA possess a slightly negative charge and have a tendency to form very thin surface layers. This property is called surface activity, and it provides the power necessary to carry substances such as toxins to the surface of the skin, intestinal tract, kidneys, and lungs where they can be removed. Although they are important and necessary to human health, the body does not produce them, so we have to ingest them.

(Seriously, the human body should come with an owner's manual.)

Gamma-linolenic acid (GLA) is an EFA in the omega-6 family and is found naturally in only a few food sources: hemp seed, black currant oil, borage oil, and evening primrose oil. The average North American diet tends to have too much omega-6 fatty acids compared to omega-3 fatty acids, because the body also converts GLA from LA, which is plentiful in cooking oil and processed foods.

For optimum health, the ratio of omega-6 to omega-3 fatty acids should be between 1:1 and 4:1. The typical North American diet is usually in the range of 11:1 to 30:1. This imbalance contributes to the development of long-term diseases such as heart disease, cancer, asthma, arthritis, and depression as well as increased risk of infection. Hemp seed oil is 55% LA and 25% LNA, or a ratio of 2.2:1; however, not all omega-6 fatty acids have the same effect on the body. Linoleic acid (not to be confused with alpha-linolenic acid, which is in the omega-3 family) and arachidonic acid (AA) promote inflammation, thereby also increasing the risk of disease, especially when consumed in excess.

In contrast, GLA actually reduces inflammation. GLA from the oils mentioned above or taken in supplement form is not converted to AA, but rather to dihomo-*gamma*-linolenic acid or DGLA. DGLA competes with AA and prevents the negative inflammatory effects that AA would otherwise cause. Having adequate amounts of certain nutrients in the body (including magnesium, zinc, and vitamins C, B3, and B6) helps promote the conversion of GLA to DGLA rather than AA, all of which hemp seed contains in significant quantities. One of the other unique things about hemp seed protein is that 65% of it is globulin edestin (from the Greek edestos or "edible"). Globulins are proteins which perform many enzymatic processes including protein synthesis and fat burning. Globulin edestin is the most readily digestible form of protein. This is good news for anybody thinking about drinking hemp protein shakes as a way to lose weight.

Legumes are another way to get beneficial protein, but don't think your meals have to be lorded over by kettles of beans. Another way to use them is to think cold sandwiches in January. There is nothing wrong with cold sandwiches in January—if they are interesting enough. You can't get much more interesting than garbanzo spread with tomato and cucumber on fresh sourdough with plantain chips on the side, even in January, although localvores might balk at the fact that tomato and cucumber aren't naturally available in January in southeast Washington State. We all have to make choices. I wish I could claim the sourdough as my own, but we are quite spoiled by our access to three very fine artisan bakeries in our area, and I am happy to pay someone else to bake my bread at this stage of life. Artisan bakeries are worth scouting out, worth the drive, and worth the cost. Good bread is life transforming, too, and once you've gotten a taste for it, you understand the grocery store variety as a deplorable, money-grubbing substitute. We like to keep cinnamon walnut loaf on hand for weekends as well as a sourdough for daily use. If we happen to be up north in Moscow, Idaho, our regional food co-op has a tempting array of organic breads, a favorite of which is the butter oat. Panhandle Artisans in Moscow also does a potato sourdough we love.

Since cooking garbanzo beans takes a few hours, I am in the habit of preparing them in large batches and freezing them. The quality and flavor are much superior to that of canned. Because of this habit, I happened to have on New Year's Day exactly four cups of cooked garbanzos in the freezer and when combined in the blender with a scallion bunch, a few cloves of garlic, a teaspoon each of basil, cumin, and oregano from the previous summer's garden, and a dollop each of mayonnaise and plain yogurt, they were downright astonishing. While we toasted the bread, we separated out just enough spread for a few sandwiches, then stirred in half a cucumber, finely chopped, and a quarter tomato, also chopped. The mix was a little mushier than I would have liked, so next time around I would relegate the tomato to slices, rather than include them in the mix. We also decided we'd like to try stirring in chopped artichoke hearts and some shredded Parmesan, maybe even pine nuts. The possibilities, as they say, are endless. As for the plantain chips, those came as a Christmas stocking-stuffer and it was the first time either of us had tried them. We were pleasantly surprised. They looked like thin slices of a large banana, were baked and lightly salted, and tasted like a potato chip. Plantains are a common food in many parts of the world and are served in the U.S. in Columbian restaurants, but are only recently being discovered here in our region. They are relatively low on the glycemic scale, thanks to their bounty of complex carbohydrates and fiber, and are dosed with plenty of Vitamin C, A, B6, folate, magnesium, and potassium. Despite being a processed food, they seemed exotic and just right for our garbanzo spread sandwiches (of which Phil had two). I decided to have mine open-faced, just so I'd have reason to double my serving of the spread. It was that satisfying and made us feel better about facing The Buffalo Dilemma.

*   *   *

We'd purchased the piece of beast the previous month in Wallowa County, Oregon. It was the product of a longstanding local buffalo ranch respected for its sustainable ranching practices and benevolent and biologically proper treatment of its herd. We literally forgot we were going vegetarian when we promised the meal to a young couple we know, and how could we back out or offer them pinto beans when they had so gleamed at the prospects of getting to try eating buffalo? No choice but to cook it anyway, eat a small amount, then send the leftovers home with them. We decided it suitable, considering the buffalo's place in indigenous North American mythology as a symbol for transformation and its prominence as a metaphor in my first novel, *Dove Creek*, which was based on my years as a public health nurse for two Pacific Northwest Indian tribes. It seemed symbolic, too, of our meeting, since Phil's office sat on the Nez Perce Indian reservation where I had once worked. And echoed a memorable moment in Phil's history, during which he was backpacking in South Dakota and woke up one morning to find a buffalo herd sleeping around him. In his words, "It made an impact on me."

So it was decided that the absolute last animal flesh either of us would ever eat was the symbolic buffalo.

This being the case, late on a Tuesday afternoon, I drained the blood off the four-ish pound chunk of buffalo flesh (you wouldn't believe how much actual blood drains out of four pounds of buffalo muscle), placed the roast in a porcelain-lined cast-iron baking dish and studded it with eight or so garlic cloves, topped it with bacon, and waited.

We seem to easily befriend people just the right age to be our children. We'd met Ben casually, through other friends, and had known him for several years. He'd done some carpentry work for us. Phil and Ben share a passion for The Grateful Dead, and we were interested to meet Kelsey, his new girlfriend (one of my daughters-in-law is also a Kelsey). But as young people will, the pair forgot about the dinner. They returned my phone message just as I was putting the roast in the oven. Our get-together was rescheduled for the next night, so I covered the meat and put it in the fridge. We were happy to make a supper of leftover lentil soup and wedges of fresh-baked, melt-in-your mouth rye bread from our local artisan bakery. We resisted the urge to eat the fudge brownies I'd also picked up from the bakery for dessert.

By six-thirty Wednesday, when they still had not arrived, Phil rang them up. Some unspecified thing had interfered. They were mortified, but they weren't going to make it.

Which was a good thing.

Because, honestly, that roast tasted terrible. The bacon turned out to be not really bacon but unflavored pork, so there wasn't the benefit of that smoky flavor. Plus, I'd either cooked it on heat too high or too low, because it was chewy and didn't separate with a fork the way I'd have liked. I was sorry I had cooked it at all.

I said a little prayer to the buffalo who had given its life as I tossed it out.

The accompanying pasta was terrible, too. I thought I could take the leftover garbanzo spread from earlier in the week, thin it with broth, lace it with a mix of Romano, Asiago, and Parmesan, throw in some basil and pine nuts, layer it over this great home-style egg pasta we get from Costco (called Country Pasta—mastering the art of home-made pasta was down the road), top it with chopped, fresh tomato, and come up with a dish worthy of guests.

Not to be. But if I were to do it again, I'd sauté two jars of artichoke hearts in butter and olive oil with a cup of mashed garbanzos, a chopped onion, toss in some pine nuts, fresh basil leaves, and a chopped tomato, and call it good. Ladle it on the pasta and top it with that shredded mix of Romano, Parmesan, and Asiago. I'd serve it with the rye bread. And I'd leave that buffalo on his hooves in Oregon.

*   *   *

One of the great things I loved about my relationship with Phil at that time was that he not only supported me to seek new horizons but he was also happy to join in my explorations with me. So it was that I happened not to be setting out on this vegetarian quest alone, as I had nineteen years prior, but with a partner and a mate. For the previous three years, the entire time Phil and I had been living together, he had done most of the cooking, because he wanted to and he was good at it. I had been too preoccupied with a writing career and making a living grading papers to care what I ate, so I mostly left the shopping and meal planning up to him.

I'm not sure how much the need for respite influenced his decision when I proposed the idea and told him I'd be doing the cooking for a while, but he seemed pretty happy about it the weekend following New Year's, sitting on the sofa watching the Texas-Alabama game while I whipped up the first batch of Oatmeal-Walnut Burgers I had made in over a decade.

Oatmeal-Walnut Burgers are one of those dishes that make you say, "Hey, this vegetarian thing isn't so bad after all!" They shouldn't look the way they do, and they shouldn't taste the way they do. Their prominent ingredients are, after all, whole oats, ground walnuts, eggs, and milk. They should look like a cookie. They should chew like a cookie. Instead, when you mince in a whole onion, add some sage, a pinch of salt, form the conglomerate into patties, brown them, then boil them for twenty-five minutes in vegetable broth, they somehow, miraculously, come out tasting pretty much like hamburgers—to my mind, anyway. We mayonnaised two slices each of fresh artisan bakery sourdough, festooned them with lettuce, dots of ketchup and mustard, slid on a patty and a slice of cheddar, and marveled. The potatoes on the side were large bakers cut into twelve slices and coated with organic sunflower oil, then sprinkled with a small amount of salt, a little cumin, and a nice helping of Tony Chachere's Original Creole Seasoning, which, by the way, makes a very nice dipping sauce if you sprinkle it into a mix of ketchup, horseradish, and mayo. It is hot, so be careful.

Cold-pressed organic sunflower oil had become my favorite cooking oil, although I'd fight you over a bottle of small-batch, artisan olive oil from certain parts of Italy. Phil and I discovered Napa Valley Naturals Organic Sunflower Oil last summer at Good Food, an organic market in Missoula, Montana. Sunflower oil is a reliable source of Vitamin E, a powerful antioxidant and anti-inflammatory considered to inhibit cancers and which we all need to power our immune functions. This particular brand is oleic sunflower oil and contains 93% monounsaturated fat and no trans-fat. It is a newer version of sunflower oil, a hybrid containing a type of linoleic acid similar to that found in hemp seed and with lower saturated fat levels than linoleic sunflower oil, which can contain up to 20% polyunsaturated fat (the semi-bad stuff). Sunflower oil of any kind benefits the cardiovascular system over, say, lard, however. Diets low in fat and high in oleic acid produce lower blood cholesterol levels, which, along with those anti-inflammatory properties, substantially decrease the risk of heart disease. The latest indications are that many chronic diseases such as heart disease, diabetes, and immune disorders are conditions that arise from constant inflammation caused by excessive amounts of animal proteins in our diets. If you think about it, our ancestors likely didn't eat a hunk of animal protein three times a day as we are used to doing. They only ate flesh when somebody's aim with a spear happened to coincide with a critter being in the wrong place at the wrong time. Studies suggest that a balanced diet in which saturated fats are replaced with sunflower oil reduces cholesterol, which is better known as the bad guy in the cholesterol/inflammation/ heart-disease drama. Cholesterol levels can actually be lowered by balancing polyunsaturated and monounsaturated fatty acids. Sunflower oil is naturally balanced in this way. Restaurants and food manufacturers are catching on to the health benefits of sunflower oil, which can be used at extremely high temperatures. It may also help food stay fresher and healthier for longer periods of time. Processed-food manufacturers, anxious to get on the health bandwagon, are using sunflower oil to replace oils containing trans-fats. Sunflower oil, like other oils, also retains moisture in the skin and may work as a barrier against infection, as well. Research involving low-birth-weight, pre-term infants (who are susceptible to infection because of their underdeveloped skin) has shown that infants receiving daily applications of sunflower oil are forty-one percent less likely to develop infections.

Phil and I had been discussing sunflower oil, among other things about our new existence, marveling in public over the sense of well-being we both had, poised over beers at our favorite brewery, the Riverport, one night later in January. In particular, one of the owners was interested in Phil's Daily Hemp Shake, as I'd decided to call it. We took a small sample of the shake to Karen and Marv, owners of the Riverport, along with an empty hemp protein can, its intact label listing the many nutritional benefits of hemp seed. We got past the usual barrage of teasing about hemp and marijuana by explaining that Phil had lost twenty-five pounds in 2009, simply by replacing his noon meal with a hemp protein shake and that I'd already begun to notice changes in my skin texture after just one week of daily shakes.

I explained to Karen that my skin texture once I started using hemp protein was noticeably different, almost a little satiny, certainly less wrinkly. Not that wrinkles are all that bad, but I was only fifty-three—too young, I mused, to be rhino-skinned. Plus, I felt lighter, more buoyant, and certainly I couldn't deny the impact on my thinking and creative impulses. The best way to put it is to say I felt more alive. I also noticed that I had more or less lost my craving for caffeine and found myself at the brewery that night drinking only a single beer (sad, but true, I know) when I might have had two. I felt like a new, improved version of my previous self.

Oh, and the best part about that Oatmeal-Walnut Burger? The recipe is for a double batch. (From *Laurel's Kitchen*, Ten Speed Press, Berkeley, 1976.)

Oatmeal-Walnut Burger

2 cups walnut pieces, ground
2 cups rolled oats
4 eggs, slightly beaten
1/2 cup skim milk
1 large onion, finely chopped
1 teaspoon sage
1/2 teaspoon salt
Fresh ground black pepper to taste
Sunflower oil
3 cups vegetable stock

Combine walnuts, oats, eggs, milk, onion, sage, salt, and pepper. Set half the mixture aside to refrigerate and save for other dishes or make the entire batch into hamburger-sized patties. Brown patties on both sides in a lightly oiled skillet, then pour the stock in around them and bring to a boil. Reduce heat and simmer, covered for 25 minutes. Serve on buns and dress as you would a beef burger, or crumble and use as you would ground beef in chili, spaghetti, etc.

Phil's Daily Hemp Shake

2 bananas or other fruit to equal 2 cups
2 heaping tablespoons hemp powder
3 heaping teaspoons plain yogurt (Nancy's Low-Fat is best)
1/2 cup (or so) fruited kefir
1/2 cup (or so) orange or other juice
1/2 cup (or so) sparkling water (we like San Pellegrino)

In a blender, chop bananas or other fruit. Add hemp powder, plain yogurt, fruited kefir, orange or other juice, and sparkling water. Adjust the ingredients to suit individual taste. Makes approximately two 16-ounce servings.

*   *   *

Phil came home from work at just before five p.m. one evening during that first month of our journey to find me in front of the computer with a bottle of sunflower oil, a jar of olives, and an open copy of *Laurel's Kitchen*. He said I looked like a wino sitting there, still in my pajamas, wearing no makeup, and my hair as askew as it had been upon awakening ten hours earlier. I laughed when I considered myself from his viewpoint and how much that sunflower oil bottle indeed looked like a wine bottle. "I just finished page twelve of our recipe book!" I told him. "I've been working all day!"

I was thankful for the opportunity to renew my relationship with *Laurel's Kitchen*. I bought it in a little bookstore in Sisters, Oregon, almost thirty years prior, not long after I had moved to the rural western U.S., a period when I felt almost no psychic kinship with anyone I knew. Reading it that first time was a form of rescue. I learned not only about vegetarian cooking and nutrition, but also about intuition, meditation, yoga, and what life was like for educated, artistic people who lived in a supportive, nonjudgmental community of others like themselves who, as Emily Dickinson put it, preferred to "dwell in possibility." At the time I had thought such a thing must exist, but I had never experienced it. These were Berkeley people, twirling the sheets in a hotbed of intellect, lunatics, and rampant artistry. I would thrive, I had always imagined, in such an environment.

A second old friend is *The Moosewood Cookbook* (Ten Speed Press, 1977), from the famous restaurant in Ithaca, New York. I have used nearly every recipe in that book, as well: Gypsy Soup, Lentil Soup, Minestrone, Russian Cabbage Borscht, Summer Vegetable Soup, Tabouli, Hummus, Pesto, Raita, Pepper and Onion Shortcake (very yummy), Stuffed Cabbage, Vegetarian Chili, Falafel, Sweet Potato Pancakes, Polenta and Spicy Vegetables, and, of course, Moosewood Fudge Brownies. You could survive a lifetime on just the recipes in *The Moosewood* and never grow bored.

Another ragged, well-loved cookbook in my kitchen is the *Follow Your Heart's Vegetarian Soup Cookbook* by Janice Cook Migliaccio. Follow Your Heart started as a small vegetarian lunch counter in Canoga

Park, California, in the 1970s. By the 1990s, several Follow Your Heart restaurants had opened and some featured organic markets. They are now the award-winning creators of Vegenaise, and they market organic salad dressings and soy-based vegan cheeses and "meat" products under the name Follow Your Heart. I don't care much for soy products for some reason, save a little tofu now and again, but you will never catch me eating anything made from soybeans that are not organic and non-GMO, now that I know that ninety percent of the U.S. soy crop is grown from Monsanto's genetically modified "Round-Up Ready" seed, thanks to a viewing of the documentary film *Food, Inc*. But my little *Follow Your Heart* cookbook has provided me with much pleasure on a few long, cold winter evenings when the snow and the wind (I sound like a Louis L'Amour novel) and the CD player were my only companions. It includes a recipe for cashew milk to use as a substitute for cow's milk in cream soups, which I have used to great results in everything from potato leek soup to corn chowder (from *Follow Your Heart's Vegetarian Soup Cookbook*, Woodbridge Press, 1983).

Cashew Milk

Blend 1-1/2 cups raw cashew pieces with 1 cup filtered water. Process in a blender until very smooth. Strain as necessary. To use as a milk substitute, add to cream soups as the very last step. Avoid boiling.

* * *

Phil wasted no time taking the plunge into vegetarian cooking and apparently had no need for a recipe book. He surprised me with lunch one Saturday—the day after he'd come home to find me hunched over the computer and the sunflower oil bottle—that featured the following little number, which had the effect of making me suspect that he was genuinely devoted to exploring this new approach to living with me. In keeping with his contracting-officer pragmatism, he used only what we had on hand.

Phil's Vegetable Roll-Ups

Mix the following ingredients together in a medium-sized bowl.

1 12-inch carrot, grated
1/4 cucumber, finely chopped
1 celery stalk, finely chopped
1/2-1 cup red cabbage, finely chopped
1/2 cup Asiago cheese, shredded
1/2 cup Romano cheese, shredded
1/2 cup Parmesan cheese, shredded
1/2 cup walnuts, finely chopped
Lettuce leaves
Tomato or spinach-flavored tortilla wraps
In a small bowl, mix the following ingredients to prepare
        the dressing.
1 cup Nancy's Plain Low-Fat Yogurt
1/4 cup Best Foods mayonnaise
2 tablespoons Annie's Organic Horseradish Mustard
1 teaspoon hot pepper sauce

Add enough dressing to the vegetable mixture to moisten it. Save any leftover dressing to thin with sunflower oil for a hot but yummy salad dressing. Spoon vegetable mixture into lettuce-lined tomato- or spinach-flavored tortilla wraps and roll into burritos.

* * *

Sometimes things don't work out as planned.

What I know now that I didn't know then is that in Phil's life, sometimes an entire late-January Saturday gets devoted to watching the first day of football playoffs instead of working on renovation projects—even if he does own a two-story 1904 Victorian just begging to have its 1980s overlay expurgated. Sometimes carpets don't get ripped from their hardwood underpinnings, decades of musty wallpaper layers don't get steamed free, the carefully crafted plaster underneath it doesn't get patched, and gallons of poetic persimmon paint don't even come close to making it to my writing studio walls.

What I know now that I didn't know then is that he can get transported to the point that he might forget to tell me his niece's college team is playing in town at six p.m. and then all of a sudden jump up and say, "Ready to go?" And that sometimes, instead of making the Cuban Picadillo recipe from *Laurel's Kitchen* from the second half of the previous Thursday night's Walnut-Oatmeal Burger recipe, I might be thankful to have that last bit of leftover garbanzo spread for whipping up a quick pair of sandwiches.

Feigning interest in sporting events burns a great number of calories, as does showing genuine interest by jumping up and down off the sofa to shout advice and exclaim over mistakes teams and players make. Many more than the few calories either of us took in that day. And then there was the need to carb-up for yard work the next day. So we gave ourselves permission that evening to splurge once again on pints—Steelhead Red Ale for me and Cedar Rock Pale Ale for him—down the road at the Riverport Brewery.

Afterwards at home, we played games of Triple Yahtzee until midnight over a bowl of agave caramel corn that didn't make us feel cotton-bodied the next morning from sugar overload.

We had no idea whether this would work, but it did, with all organic ingredients, and beautifully. As for the butter with its solid block of saturated fats, well, life is all about balance, and nobody's perfect, and using real butter is right up there with putting actual cream in my coffee—an occasional pleasure I find no need to justify or change.

Agave Caramel Corn

1/2 cup organic popcorn kernels
1 tablespoon sunflower oil
2 tablespoons canola oil
1/2 cup agave syrup
1/2 cup butter
1/2 teaspoon baking soda

Preheat oven to 300 degrees. Butter two cookie sheets. Place oil and several corn kernels into a heavy-bottomed kettle on a moderately high flame. Heat until test kernels pop, then add the rest of the popcorn and cover with a lid. Shake pan over heat until corn popping slows to a rate of 1 every 5 seconds. Divide popped corn between two doubled, full-sized brown paper grocery sacks and set aside. In a medium-sized saucepan, heat agave syrup and butter to a rolling boil and cook for 3-4 minutes. Turn off heat. Add baking soda and stir into hot liquid. The mixture will turn foamy. Drizzle 1/8 cup at a time over popped corn, intermittently closing grocery sacks and shaking to distribute foam and coat corn evenly. Divide coated corn between the two baking sheets and spread out evenly. Bake at 300 degrees for 5 minutes then remove from oven and stir. Return to oven for 5 more minutes then remove from oven and stir again. Repeat this process until corn is golden brown. Allow to cool before eating. Be very careful since the hot agave mixture can cause severe burns.

*   *   *

For breakfast on a Monday morning a person can do worse than to eat leftover-from-the-weekend Skillet Cakes made with hemp, spelt, and oats, alongside a Pumpkin Pudding. The amount of fiber in those two things alone is about ten grams. The fiber in a quart of Phil's Daily Hemp Shake comes to about fifteen grams. That's five grams short of the minimum recommended daily total. Add two big bowls of Moosewood's Gypsy Soup for dinner, which is nothing but vegetables and beans, which are pretty much nothing but fiber, and you'll be the Fiber Champion of the Day.

Adjusting to a high-fiber diet takes time. Since Phil went down into the mine first, so to speak (he'd been drinking daily hemp shakes for a year), I consulted him. "Trust me," he said. "It gets better." (This is the man who, when I expressed my consternation over the buffalo dilemma said, "Well, buffalo are vegetarian.") To myself, I was thinking, *we're talking ecclesiastical peeing and pooping here. It's been ten days. I'm burning more calories than I'm taking in just running to the bathroom!*

The problem, of course, was not what I was eating *now* but what I had been eating *before*. Even though I'd primarily followed an organic diet for most of my adult life, and fairly religiously, suffice it to say there were plenty of processed items in the organic foods section of nearly every grocery store and with a local rancher having opened up a meat market less than a mile away, and having lived for the last three years with Phil cooking dishes day and night from meat, sausage, poultry, fish, and, obviously, buffalo—well, surely I needed to expect it might take some time for things to catch up with themselves. Some of that stuff, beef in particular, works its way out of the body over a period of days and perhaps—as some postulate—weeks. The human body is actually pretty inefficient at digesting muscle fiber, which is why intestinal cancer is more common in cultures where animals are the prominent source of protein. We evolved over the eons as hunters and gatherers. Animal meat was available rarely enough that its acquisition was celebrated, and a man's worth was measured by his ability to kill for the group. Rituals to bless the hunt evolved for a reason: if you went out and burned all those calories trying to kill something, you darned well better kill something. Most of what many of our very recent ancestors ate was grown or gathered. In my family, the number of quart jars of beans and vegetables dwarfed considerably what was hanging in the smokehouse. And you didn't butcher a chicken unless it was for company or a special occasion. Beans and eggs and what grew in the garden, that's what people from my part of the world ate.

More and more I am convinced this is what our bodies wish we all ate. And I believe it's possible that even depression arises from our failure to fuel our bodies correctly. But the reason for the bloating and diarrhea is that our twenty-first century small intestine has grown lazy. It is not used to being asked to work at a snappy pace, which fiber requires of it. It is like a body on welfare: accustomed to the slow, slogging drudgery of pretending—pretending to be concerned with laboring.

In other words, in the human gut, breaking down animal flesh to its protein components and then to amino acids requires very little physical effort on the part of the intestine. But the problem is, the intestine is actually healthiest when it is working the hardest. It's no secret that unused muscle goes slack, grows lazy. We all know how hard it is to get up and start working out when we've let ourselves get out of shape.

In the case of the small intestine, it becomes too lazy to even process water and siphon it to the kidney, so any excess water—processing animal flesh requires very little of it—just sort of creeps out of the intestine and into the tissues.

Yes, you heard it here: eating animal protein makes you bloat. Fiber sucks water into itself. It can't get enough of the stuff. It vacuums fluid right out of your tissues so it can be routed through the kidneys (oh heavenly days for the kidneys, which love this kind of work) and made into urine. (Hence the peeing.) Other kinds of fiber are cholesterol magnets. They cart the lousy, villainous goop right out of the body and flush it straight to the deep blue sea. This is the cartoon version of how this all works, but hopefully the idea is clear.

Skillet Cakes, by the way, are a high-powered pancake I came up with for Sunday breakfast. They remind me of buckwheat, which are my favorite. But be careful to use a low flame. High heat destroys Omega-3s in hemp protein and the cakes are thick enough that they take a bit of time to cook through. Warm up leftovers by toasting them on low in the toaster. And the Pumpkin Pudding was an adaptation of a Pumpkin Flan recipe I found in Sunday's *Parade*. It was a perfect breakfast sweet.

Skillet Cakes

> 1 cup unbleached white flour
> 1 cup spelt flour
> 1 cup oat flour
> 1 teaspoon baking soda
> 2 heaping tablespoons hemp powder
> 1 teaspoon cardamom
> 1/2 cup sunflower oil
> 1/2 cup milk
> 1/2 cup plain yogurt
> 2 eggs
> 1 cup sparkling mineral water

In a large bowl, mix together all three flours. Stir in the baking soda, hemp powder, and cardamom. In a separate small bowl, combine the sunflower oil, milk, yogurt, and eggs. Pour the liquid mixture into the dry mixture. Add enough sparkling mineral water to make a thick batter. Cook on oiled griddle over low heat until browned on both sides and cooked through.

Pumpkin Pudding

1 15-ounce can of pumpkin
3 large egg yolks
2 large eggs
1/3 cup agave syrup, plus more for drizzling
1/3 cup plain yogurt
1 8-ounce carton vanilla bean yogurt
Butter for coating ramekins

Blend the pumpkin, egg yolks, eggs, syrup, and yogurt in a food processor until very smooth. Coat six 6-ounce heatproof ramekins with butter. Bake at 350 degrees for 30 minutes. Let cool. Run a butter knife blade around inside edges of ramekins and unmold puddings onto plates. Drizzle with agave syrup and dollop with vanilla bean yogurt.

WAXING GIBBOUS MOON

WITH NEWS OF DISASTER in another part of the world, it was hard to think about how we'd been voluntarily restricting food intake those first few weeks of 2010, snug in the cozy period warmth of our 104-year-old Victorian home, when so many mind-boggling numbers were suffering in Haiti from one of the worst earthquakes in anyone's memory. Hard to place too much importance on our first restaurant foray as vegetarians—the way Phil dialed the phone number to Thai Garden down the street, the way the proprietress knew who he was from the sound of his voice and the fact that he asked for no mushrooms. "No mussooms," she always says, in the form of a greeting, this Tic Tac® of a Thai woman who gets so excited about seeing us she claps her hands each time we step through the door. It was tough, twirling my fork into slick rice noodles and peppered green beans, eating the sweet-crusted, deep-fried tofu, stopping to take breaths between the heat of three-stars worth of red chili seed, to keep from feeling unworthy of the level of ease with which I had lived out the day. It was painful to think about having *chosen* to make a meal out of toast the previous night. It was hard to think of anything but those people in Haiti.

My friend, writer and radio producer Jill Nugent, had been going to Haiti every year for almost a decade, coming back with her graying dreadlocks modified by village women. She went there to teach farming methods and help plant gardens. The daughter of upper-middle-class Ohioans and the former wife of a fancy Cleveland attorney, for more than thirty years she had lived the Western immigrant story in a real way, growing and raising practically everything she and her family needed, chasing milk goats, blowing breath into baby chickens, surviving insane odds with a moody, abusive, alcoholic, frontier artist, and Idaho Panhandle winters in sturdy but primitive homes. Fifty-nine at the time of this writing, Jill still grows most of what she eats. She raises sheep to make wool, which she then spins by hand into yarn for sweaters, socks, mittens, and hats. She gathers and dries wild herbs and knows how to use them, knows what each one treats. I cured my earaches with mullein leaf tea on her advice. It works, and it's cheaper than a doctor visit and easier on the body than antibiotics.

Her house is built into her part of a mountain just outside of Moscow, Idaho, and the inside of it is always hung with drying things: clothes racks full of yarn dyed in every color with a fungus she has shipped from New Zealand; berries, tomatoes, and apples spread out on old window screens suspended from the ceiling; hanks of herbs, chilis, and garlic. She cooks and cans and bakes on a wood cook range. Serves up soup from pots simmered on her barrel-bellied wood heater. Has to plot and plan ways to drive off the moose. Can't grill salmon outside because it attracts bears. Produces her own electricity with a squadron of batteries wired to an array of solar panels. She is not vegetarian but knows the pedigree of just about everything she puts into her mouth and is otherwise the best and most inventive cook I've ever known. I asked for permission to include her recipe for The World's Best Granola, but she said, "Why don't you include the recipe for your version of the World's Best Granola?" What follows is from an email she sent shortly after the earthquake in Haiti:

"Most of the news from the media is coming from the capital and other cities where the situation is very bad. Most construction is of concrete that is skimpy on cement and rebar. (Once I heard a homeowner argue with a handyman over whether a repair was going to require four or six nails.) The poorest people live in shacks made of materials propped together. In the cities, the destruction, terror, and suffering going on now are on a scale that is hard for us to imagine. Survivors won't have access to clean water; sanitation will go south; the roads that bring food from the countryside are surely broken and every family has lost loved ones. The disaster on LaGonave has a somewhat different flavor. Casualties and damage are less in the countryside than in the capital. Life is lived outdoors. There are fewer buildings and fewer people inside them. They experienced shock after shock. Many houses fell down. People were hurt, but I don't know that anyone was killed. People are frantic for family members on the mainland, especially children going to high school in Port au Prince. Cracked cisterns will cause water shortages. The transportation system that brings food to the island—docks, roads, vehicles, ships, and boats—is entirely disrupted, so in a few days there will start to be a critical food shortage there. The good news/bad news is that the progressive community on LaGonave has experience with this kind of catastrophe—in the aftermath of the coup of 2004 and the hurricanes of 2008, they faced crises of similar magnitude (from which they are still recovering). Even now they are organizing their response. There will be a fund to expand school meal programs to include families. They might charter a boat to bring food over from the mainland. They will know what to do. There will be a fund to expand the reconstruction program put together after the hurricanes. More good news is a coalition of groups called "Farming is Life." They have been working for many years to heal environmental damage and strive for food sustainability. Every year they make gains towards the goal of making the island less vulnerable to these kinds of food crises. LaGonave is a remote hinterland of Haiti, so help that emanates from the capital might or might not trickle there."

Paula's Version of the World's Best Granola

8 cups nuts of any kind
1/2 stick butter, melted
1/2 cup agave syrup
1 16-ounce jar orange marmalade
4 tablespoons vanilla
1/2 teaspoon sea salt
16 cups oats
Dried fruit, amount and type as preferred

Preheat oven to 200 degrees. Chop nuts in food processor. Make a liquid of butter, agave, marmalade, 1-2 cups water, vanilla, and salt. Bring to a boil. Place nuts in a very large pan and pour liquid over them. Stir. Add oats and mix. Pay attention to dryness level and add water to liquid mix if it looks like you are going to need it. Don't get it too wet. Spread evenly over as many ungreased cookie sheets as your oven will hold (I can get four in mine). Toast for one hour, then begin checking every 15 minutes until granola is very dark but not yet burning (in other words, slightly over-toast the mix). This may take as long as 2 hours. Stir in dried fruit after granola has cooled. Store, well-sealed, in a cool, dark place.

*   *   *

I tried to make sense of this against a bourgeois backdrop of self-induced hunger accompanied by an inability to concentrate. The problem was that after weeks of subsisting on plant protein and fiber and almost no fat, I was hungry all the time, even though I hadn't kept any of my promises to get up early and walk in the mornings. Instead I drove the fifteen blocks, a guilty-as-charged American, to the coffee shop in my pajamas, same as always, for a single-tall-extra-cream double-shot Americano.

The solution sounded simple: stop complaining or eat more.

But what?

Phil came up with the idea to boil some eggs, and I always tried to keep yogurt in the fridge, but boiled eggs and yogurt had to be kept cool, more aforethought and preparation than I would ever be able to muster in the mornings. We both needed something packable and storable with a dose of protein because, of course, we'd already figured out that neither of us was getting quite enough. The problem for me was being back in the classroom after the holiday break and realizing just exactly how much energy a person burns teaching a pair of seventy-five-minute college writing classes a day. Before, the solution was simply to go have another cup of coffee. Now I understood I had been operating on adrenalin and caffeine, which eventually was going to take its toll, and in fact, already was in the form of disrupted sleep. What was happening was that I came into my morning class charged from, say, a bowl of fruit and oatmeal, but the hemp shake wasn't keeping me going through the afternoon. Phil and I discussed this, because he was coming home hungry as a Venus flytrap, and he acted like one, too, snapping at anything that spoke or came too close.

At the same time, we were talking about the sense of extreme well-being we both had, and the effect the change in routine was having on our appetites overall. We both admitted that sometimes the feeling was not so much hunger, rather a feeling of needing something. Phil said, "One thing about going vegetarian is that you end up not eating because you realize you really don't need very much, as long as it's the right type of food you are eating to begin with." We both agreed that the "something" we felt was the feeling that we should be eating, but on closer examination felt like we didn't truly need to. We were, gross as it sounds, used to filling our time with eating. Eating as entertainment. The realization made me feel even worse. Perhaps as evidence, two nights prior Phil had been pining (read groaning) for a hamburger and threatening to eat meat while I was out of town the next week. The exchange reminded me of my dilemma and solution when I was trying to raise my pre-adolescent sons as vegetarians: Protein Balls. Protein Balls (adapted from *Laurel's Kitchen*) each have about 100 calories, 5 grams of protein, and maybe 2 grams of fiber each. They are awesome and addictive, especially if you dip them in melted carob chips, and are the perfect stand-in for candy and granola bars. I've adapted the recipe to accommodate the hemp powder and agave syrup.

Protein Balls

2 cups almond or peanut butter
1/3 cup toasted wheat germ
4 tablespoons hemp powder
1/2 cup skim milk powder (the health-food store kind, not the
        regular kind—two different animals)
1/3 cup agave syrup
1/2 cup dried currants
1/4 cup dried cranberries, chopped
1/4 cup sunflower seeds, chopped
1/2 teaspoon sea salt
1 12-ounce bag carob chips
2 tablespoons butter

In a large bowl, mix nut butter, wheat germ, milk powder, hemp powder, agave syrup, currants, cranberries, sunflower seeds, and salt. Add extra milk powder as needed to create a moldable but not sticky dough. Roll mixture into 1-inch balls or press onto a flat surface until it is 1/2 inch thick then cut into 1-1/2 inch squares. In a small pan over low heat, melt carob and butter and stir. Dip balls or squares into melted carob and butter mixture. Place balls or squares on wax paper and allow to rest until coating is set before eating. Store in the refrigerator for up to two weeks.

*   *   *

One way to escape TV football is to find something else to do. And what could be better than going on a road trip by myself for a family gathering in Boise? The experience also gave me occasion to review my reasons for deciding to return to a vegetarian lifestyle:

- I get to stare at my organic cottage cheese and organic salad while the rest of the family eats non-organic, baked, bone-in ham and non-organic au gratin potatoes made with non-organic cream of chicken soup.

- I get to explain how dairy products don't have souls.

- I get to explain how eating an egg is not the same as butchering a chicken.

- I get to explain how eating low on the food chain and choosing organically produced foods supports small and local farmers and helps send the message that we care about what we put into our bodies and that we are on to the weirdoes in government and the corporations who don't care if they're making us sick since they are also the ones making money off of so-called "health care."

- I get to explain how methane from cattle production contributes significantly to the ozone layer's destruction.

- I get to explain how not buying a pound of ground beef saves two thousand gallons of water.

- I get to explain how I get my protein from hemp seed, legumes, grains, nuts, eggs, and yogurt.

- I get to explain how eating beans regularly is the best way to prevent them from causing flatus.

- I get to explain how hemp seed is not marijuana.

- I get to explain how alive I feel.

- I get to explain how my cholesterol went from 150 to 220 after a decade of eating meat and how the simple act of eating a bowl of oatmeal each morning for a month dropped it to 200 and how you eventually stop having diarrhea from all that fiber.

- I get to explain that I lost 125 pounds during the first year the first time I became a vegetarian and kept it off for a decade.

- I get to explain how I gained 110 pounds as an omnivore in the subsequent decade.

- I get to explain how loose my clothes feel after only two weeks.

- I get to order homemade apple pie at Idaho restaurants while travelling to Boise to meet my brand-new granddaughter because it's the only thing on the menu that doesn't contain meat. Unless you count a grilled Velveeta sandwich.

* * *

This particular family gathering was more than just an escape, however, it was the precious introduction to a new grandbaby. Of course it was also a source of consternation and hard work, since somebody had to feed everyone. There were two of us grandmothers on hand to share the kitchen and help in the aftermath of my son Sean and his wife Susannah having presented to the world their second daughter, little Leah, or "Lady Bug" as we immediately began calling her. My and Gwen's styles marked either ends of the cooking continuum: she in her very early seventies and the traditionalist; I, the free-spirited one, in my mid-life vegetarian rebirth. Since by the second night I had declared it my turn to cook, we were at the Boise Co-op in search of the ingredients for Lasagna al Forno, an old favorite from *Laurel's Kitchen* and always a reliable crowd-pleaser.

Food co-ops as we know them now have been around since the 1960s, although cooperative food buying dates back much earlier. I have belonged to food co-ops consistently since 1979, when I joined the First Alternative Food Co-op in Corvallis, Oregon. It was an hour's drive from where I was living, but it was worth the effort once a month to drive down and stock up on oats, flour, honey, fresh-ground peanut butter, torula yeast, milk powder, seeds, nuts, cheeses, carob chips, and bulk spices. They also sold exotic items such as incense and natural sponges, handmade soap, earth-scented coffee beans, baskets, and batiks. They were the closest things to open-air markets at the time, and I loved the shaggy-hippy people with their Zen attitudes who volunteered to cut cheese from plate-sized wheels and ring up customer purchases. Both my sons grew up shopping with me in co-ops, and now I was introducing my thirty-two-month-old granddaughter Malory to them, as well as her "other" grandmother, who only looked at me slightly askew when I purchased fresh local greenhouse spinach, organic walnuts, and expensive organic Roma tomatoes from Mexico for the sauce. (I prefer to purchase what is local and in season as much as possible, but this had to be perfect, so canned tomatoes wouldn't do. Plus there is that "thing" about the acid from canned tomatoes leaching something out of their tin housing we'd rather not know about.) I also splurged on whole-milk mozzarella instead of part-skim. (A word of warning is due here, because once you try the former, you will never again settle for the latter.) We cruised the aisle with Malory seated in the cart, clutching a bouquet of daisies she wanted to purchase for her mother "because it's such a special day." This being the first time the three of us had gone on an adventure alone together, the two grandmothers had to agree. "Can you believe it?" Malory said at one point to a passing fellow customer, "I have two grandmothers!"

Lasagna al Forno is particularly close to my heart because I discovered it on the same day in 1980 that I discovered *Laurel's Kitchen*, at the home of some university folks in Corvallis, Oregon, two months before I delivered the son who twenty-something years later fathered first Malory, then Leah. I have cooked and canned gallons of the sauce and tweaked it over the years until it has become my own. The spinach and the chopped, toasted walnuts create a texture so sufficiently comparable to meat that no one ever misses it—save my youngest son, Jacob, who for some strange reason eschews nuts altogether. I have also used tofu in this recipe, in the days before the GMO catastrophe. It helps to use the firmer varieties and freeze it first, which, once thawed, gives it a texture close to ground meat. I have not yet added hemp powder to the sauce, but there is no reason not to, keeping in mind that the oven must then be kept below 350 degrees, lest the omegas be destroyed.

Dinner, by the way, was a great success.

Paula's Lasagna al Forno

Sauce:

1/4 cup olive oil
2 medium red onions, chopped
4 cloves garlic, mashed
1 bell pepper, chopped
3 carrots, grated
3 bay leaves
1 tablespoon oregano
2 teaspoons thyme
1 tablespoon basil
2 teaspoons rosemary
2 teaspoons fennel
1/2 cup dried parsley
2 tablespoons paprika
6 cups chopped fresh tomatoes
2 6-ounce cans tomato paste
1 teaspoon fresh ground black pepper
2 tablespoons agave syrup
Vegetable broth

Sauté onion, garlic, and pepper in olive oil over medium heat until onion just begins to caramelize. Stir in carrots and herbs and cook until pungent, about another 10-15 minutes. Add tomatoes, tomato paste, black pepper, and agave syrup. Thin with broth as needed. Cover and simmer for 20-30 minutes.

Lasagna:

1 sauce recipe
1 pound DeBoles' Organic Jerusalem Artichoke Lasagna Noodles
1 quart whole milk ricotta cheese
2 cups toasted walnuts, chopped
8 ounces grated Asiago cheese
2 bunches fresh spinach, chopped
1 pound whole milk mozzarella cheese

Preheat oven to 325 degrees. Spread a layer of sauce on the bottom of a Dutch oven. (Baking dishes are too shallow.) Lay enough dry lasagna noodles on top of sauce to cover it. Spread half the ricotta on top of the noodles for the next layer. Top with 1/3 of the nuts, and 1/4 of the Asiago. Add another layer of sauce, then another layer of noodles, making sure the noodles run the opposite direction of the first layer. Spread spinach over the noodles and top with sliced mozzarella, saving enough to grate for the top. Add another layer of sauce, then more noodles, again, changing the direction the noodles run. Spread the rest of the ricotta on the noodles next and another 1/3 of the nuts. Add a final layer of noodles in the other direction, then more sauce. Top with the rest of the mozzarella, grated, and the rest of the nuts. Cover with foil held in place by the Dutch oven lid. Bake for one hour. Let sit covered for 30 minutes before serving.

* * *

When I was about fourteen years old, my family suddenly decided to leave the American Baptist Church in favor of the Assembly of God. Overnight we went from being normal, sane, poor, working-class people to being what some people refer to as Holy Rollers. I spent my teenage years watching people speaking in tongues, dancing in the Spirit, laying on hands for healing, being "slain" in the Spirit, and—to fit in, I now understand—engaging in these things myself.

I have since come to think of the Holy Spirit as the human creative spirit. I like to think I am engaging this Spirit each time I turn away from following a recipe in a cookbook in favor of following my own instincts. In fact, I've worked very hard to develop my sense of intuition by practicing exercises shared with me during the years I worked as a community health nurse with Northwest Indian tribes. One thing I was instructed to do was to try to discern who is calling before answering the phone, which is why to this day I do not have caller ID. Another trick is to concentrate on lowering your center of gravity, focus on your lower central gut region, as you do when skiing. Eastern thought calls this the *qi*, the center of a human from which life energy radiates. Indigenous people don't spend much time in their heads. They live their lives by learning to sense from their guts. Coming from Cherokee and African heritage gave me a leg up, and my mother and sister both have similar abilities. My sister Traci, in fact, has dreamed of murders before they've happened, although she can never get the police to believe her. My mother's predictions are becoming less accurate as she gets older, but when she tells me about her dreams, I listen. And I do sometimes sense something before it happens, either that or I'll dream it, but I only seem to recognize the precognition in retrospect. Still, this vague ability has served me well in some very strange ways, and I've learned to pay closer attention to that still, quiet voice. More than once I have gotten into my car in a mildly transcendent state, only to find myself at a book store or antique store and then walking straight in to buy whatever was calling me; and in the case of books, it is usually the exact piece of research I need for whatever writing project I'm working on. Phil and I both have this odd ability, and our home is filled with items we've acquired in this way. It is, I suppose, just as with our cooking, an art form. Although I still cannot consistently tell who's calling before I pick up the phone.

One particular dark day in 1997, full of doubt about my chosen career as a writer and walking the soaked streets of Moscow, Idaho, with a clear sense of feeling drawn toward *something* but having no inkling of what that might be, I decided chasing intuition was a bunch of bunk and slouched home in the rain. Five minutes later, unable to let go of the sense of being pulled in a particular direction, I got in my car and drove to a local antique store. I parked, entered the store, and walked straight to the back to find a copy of *The Art of Intuition* by Virginia Burden. Long since out of print, the book explains intuition's role in the concept of theosophy (from the Greek *theosophia* or god-wisdom), which is the notion that a universal spiritual hierarchy exists to help humanity on its evolutionary path, one person at a time, and that our instinctual perception of this has led us to formulate religions. The *Oxford English Dictionary* describes it as, "Any system of speculation which bases the knowledge of nature upon that of the divine nature." Burden's book made me understand the human sense of intuition as our link to our natural selves and the natural world. For a while I became obsessed with trying to understand intuition and its purpose in human existence. Years, in fact. What I discovered is that a honed intuition is a necessary tool for a poet and a writer— the best, as it turns out—and that following intuition, or "gut feelings," is an authentic approach to research. What emerges in the writing is an organic experience for both the writer and the reader.

It was this brand of instinct that led me to buy French green lentils at the Boise Co-op that same day, only to later read about their immense nutritional power. I've always enjoyed the various types of lentils, more than once having proclaimed after eating a bowl of lentil soup that I had been nourished in my soul. They were a staple in my first vegetarian incarnation. More recently, having lived nearly twenty years in the Palouse region of the Inland Northwest, the lentil capital of the U.S., I have come to think of lentils as commonplace, even though most Americans are not overly fond of them, and you can't exactly find them on a McDonald's menu board. Perhaps it is because every autumn, Pullman, Washington, where I teach English at a state university, hosts the annual Lentil Festival, at which everything from lentil chili to lentil ice cream and lentil-zucchini bread can be sampled. Lentils have long been considered "poor man's meat," although many have praised their qualities, and it is thought they may have once been used as currency. Perhaps it is this association with the lowly that has bestowed on them their ability to benefit the spirit as well as the body.

The earliest lentils were found in Greece, dating back to 13,000 B.C.E., and in Syria and Palestine at about 8,000 B.C.E. Esau in the Christian Bible gave up his birthright for a dish of lentils (Genesis 25:30-34). Pliny wrote about medicinal uses for lentils. Hippocrates prescribed them to his patients for liver ailments. Nutritionists recommend them as a substitute for meat because gram for gram their protein content is thirty percent greater than beef. One cup of boiled lentils also provides 38 milligrams of calcium, 356 milligrams of phosphorus, 72 milligrams of magnesium, 360 micrograms of folic acid, 6.6 milligrams of iron, 731 milligrams of potassium, and 10 grams of fiber. They can be sprouted and added to salads for a protein boost, or ground in a food processor, made into patties, and used like burger. *Laurel's Kitchen* has a recipe for Lentil Nut Loaf so tasty and rich it needs nothing but a salad to accompany it. I used the French green lentils to create the best lentil soup I've ever made, at least the portion I ate. I can't speak to the larger pot of it to which I added leftover ham for the rest of the family.

Herbed French Lentil Soup

1/4 cup olive oil
2 red onions, finely chopped
2 carrots, grated
6 cloves garlic, coarsely chopped
2 bay leaves
1/4 cup dried parsley
1 teaspoon ground rosemary
1 teaspoon dried basil
1 teaspoon fresh ground pepper

1 teaspoon sea salt
Dash of cayenne
4 cups vegetable broth
2 cups organic French green lentils
8 cups water

Sauté onion, carrots, and garlic in olive oil until onion is transparent. Add spices. Add broth and lentils. Add water. Bring to boil. Simmer uncovered over low heat for 1 hour or until lentils are soft. Serve with pita wedges and hummus or homemade cheese.

*   *   *

Some years ago I journeyed to magical British Columbia with my friends Kathy and Patty to attend what they described as a "Wise Woman Retreat," at which I had agreed to read from my first poetry chapbook. It is true that I am now a university English instructor, but I am also trained as a registered nurse with a significant history as a public health nurse. Patty, Kathy, and I had all been working for the Coeur d'Alene tribe in Plummer, Idaho. Kathy was a clinic nurse; Patty was a nurse practitioner; and I oversaw community health programs. It was my thirty-eighth birthday, and my last day on the job. My team of nurses and nursing assistants and I had designed the first public health program on an Indian reservation to serve both Indian and non-Indian clients. They had all received national awards, and I, as a commissioned officer with the U.S. Public Health Service, had been decorated. I still have the small, striped bar that was meant to be worn on my Navy-issue uniform. The goal was to celebrate my separation from the USPHS and my decision to become a writer. Six months prior, I had given notice of my resignation and the surrendering of my commission.

British Columbia in September is dreamy, with crayon-blue skies and foliage tricked out in the shades of autumn. The air snipped at me and I didn't mind, reminding me as it did of the inhalation of each breath. Patty, Kathy, and I wound our way up a mountain road to a wilderness lake and camp, talking about the intoxicating scenery, the mysteries of life, and the stop we had made at a winery to sample iced champagne.

The retreat turned out to be a gathering of Wicca practitioners. Pagans. The exact opposite of Christian fundamentalism. We were all sworn not to reveal our activities to the outside world, but I am here to tell you that the drumming circle pulled a thunderstorm from a sky star-laden enough to navigate the seas, and the packed earth of the great assembly shelter shifted while the walls trembled from the accompanying winds.

But I was less impressed with that than I was with the savory, fresh, organic, vegetarian fare and the express assertion by conference organizers that good, natural food was everyone's first priority. The second night, after a meal of soup, hummus, homemade bread, and a soul-stopping dessert called "Death by Chocolate" (which I can only describe as a tumbled combination of cake, brownie, and pudding—again, all organic, not too sweet, and a bona fide drug), I held my poetry reading in front a medieval-sized fireplace and a room packed with physically fit women of all colors, ages, and sizes, all buzzing from the chocolate and cups of coffee. I was so glad to see that no wine came out. No alcohol of any kind. Those women didn't need it.

Had I never understood the power of the feminine before, I did then. The potential in the room was hugely palpable. It raised the hair on my arms and filtered through me like champagne bubbles.

Although I used my time and inspiration at the retreat for writing rather than attending "witchy" workshops, I did succumb to a Tarot reading—which predicted I would find true love, live my life as a writer, and find happiness after a long stretch of difficulty—and a Reike treatment which left me feeling buoyant and youthful. At one point I also attended a "Naming Circle" meant to reveal to us our representative icon. Perhaps thirty of us stood in a large ring around a high priestess who walked the inner circle, facing each of us, stopping briefly and declaring to the crowd and the world our single defining characteristic.

Mine was fire.

Once the naming was finished, we each traveled, one at a time, the same path the high priestess had walked, "sharing" our named energy with other participants by "sending" our energy out towards them. In the last moments of the ceremony, she revealed to us what she described as her single most important message: Avoid processed food. "It contains the death crystals," she said, "and will rob you of your power." That sentence finds its way to my forebrain on a very regular basis even still, almost two decades later, and became so predominant in my thoughts at the end of 2009 that I couldn't ignore it. For years I have started New Year's with a three-day fast, a ritual of renewal I learned from a Nez Perce friend. As I prepared myself in mind and spirit for the beginning of 2010, the urge to return to a vegetarian lifestyle came with it.

These words also haunted me during my stay at my son's in Boise as day after day we contemplated what to prepare for dinner. My dear daughter-in-law Susannah one afternoon admitted with profound apology that she craved beef; this for the first time in nine months. Throughout her pregnancy she was unable to tolerate the smell of meat, whether raw, cooked, or refrigerated. Privately, I considered the possibility of the gestating fetus's ability to protect itself from growth hormones and cow antibiotics by generating the whims of the pregnant mother. (Of, course, we now know, almost three years later, little Leah was a born vegetarian. She refuses meat entirely. Won't touch it.)

And so I stood quietly by as my son and I shopped for a meal at Walmart. He had been laid off from his web designer job for a year. Walmart, he explained when I protested, is part of how they were surviving. I bit my tongue at the eight-dollar package of overly red ground beef product, wanting badly to say that three pounds of organic legumes would be less than half of that. And so the family ate burgers made from that two-pound package of Walmart ground beef, which contained so much dye that despite cooking the meat until it was almost too dry to eat, it remained pink. I was thankful for my un-dyed leftover Herbed French Lentil Soup and my open-faced cheese and tomato sandwich on potato bread from the Boise Co-op. At the very least, everyone came to the conclusion that they would no longer purchase meat from Walmart. I wished I could convince them to stop shopping there, period. It worried me, their dependence on food that came preformed and conformed. Although it didn't happen all the time, Malory lunched occasionally on dinosaur-shaped chicken nuggets, which we now know come from a meat by-product called "pink slime," and breakfasted on pancakes from a freezer bag. And one midday, a kiddie TV dinner.

At least I could rest knowing baby Leah, for some time to come, was privy to her mother's milk—the last perfect food any of us gets to consume.

*   *   *

Thanks to the wonders of technology, I left Boise with two CDs full of photos of Malory and Leah. I toted home my jar of hemp powder, the bottle of agave syrup, the organic rice cakes, the organic whole oats, the sparkling mineral water, the kefir, and the plain yogurt. I left the organic onions and carrots and spinach and apples because I knew they would get used. I also carried the memories and warm feelings one has from such a week and one gray, sad secret: on that final day, I ate meat.

It was an accident.

We had decided to scavenge for dinner since we each became hungry at our own pace after an afternoon of burgers (again) at Five Guys Burgers (grilled tomato and cheese for me, again) and, heaven forbid, donuts from a place called Country Donuts (mine was a single chocolate-frosted buttermilk bar I shall never forget). Sean and I had made brilliant pizzas completely from scratch the night before, and while he was busy loading photos from the various cameras to CDs for Gwen and me to cart home, with Gwen, Susannah, and Leah looking on, I decided to warm up leftover slices for everyone. More cheese, more tomatoes, more bread.

Perhaps I should have turned on the lights in the kitchen when I decided to retrieve a slice, but likely you can guess what happened. I had walked back into the living room where the rest of the family were munching on various food items and was halfway into that first slice before I realized that what I was tasting was not merely spicy sauce but pepperoni and Canadian bacon camouflaged and buried under cheese, olives, and tomatoes. I kept my discovery to myself because I didn't want to endure the teasing, stood there by the counter separating the living room and kitchen and finished the last bites. I could have silently walked to the pantry and thrown it in the trash but was afraid someone would question it. Pretty silly, I know, and it made me feel very, very sad. It felt, well, like a little death.

But it also tasted *so good.*

And yet, being characteristically guilt-ridden as I am, it was the little death feeling that dogged me for the entire return trip home. Once there, however, I found quick salvation in those photos. I looked happy and comfortable with myself and my surroundings. As the "other" grandma Gwen said when I'd first arrived, I was "sparkling from the inside out," and I looked like someone who knew it. It kept occurring to me that in returning to a vegetarian lifestyle, I had unearthed some forgotten truth about myself. Being a vegetarian was not just a skin I was trying on. What I came to understand was that I was—also characteristically, perhaps—neither carnivore nor omnivore.

It was not a religion but a truth. A truth and a belief that not consuming meat was and is important to my well-being. To the well-being, perhaps, of all of us here in America.

And to the well-being of the entire earth community.

* * *

Thank goodness for Subway where they sell toasted flatbread topped with jalapeno jack, lettuce, tomato, red onion, green pepper, spinach, cucumber, banana peppers, and a very thin line of Chipotle Southwestern sauce—a very passable vegetarian road meal that's easily handled behind the wheel. This little bit of aforethought allowed me to take a shortcut west of Boise off the I-84 freeway into Oregon that looped back around through scenic snow-harnessed farmland to Weiser, landing me at Phil's office on the west end of the Nez Perce reservation in just four hours and twenty minutes. That's with no potty breaks. It boarded off the hunger pangs until I sat down with Phil over a plate of vegetarian Confetti Nachos at Rooster's Landing in Clarkston.

Back at the house, a game of Triple Yahtzee afterward was enough to send both of us searching for comfort food before we started the second game (and yes, I did wonder about the relationship between those table games and our craving for treats, or was it simply a celebration of reunion?) and that led us to invent Banana-Peach Crunch, which was nothing but a variation of that Midwest favorite, Banana Pudding. Varying the ingredients might end in disappointment, and since the brands are readily available at food co-ops, health food stores, and supermarkets with natural foods sections, there's no reason not to seek them out. I'd say make a double batch, but it doesn't keep, and it's too rich to eat more than a serving. Definitely not breakfast fare.

Banana-Peach Crunch

2 medium organic bananas
1 1/2 cups Nature's Path Organic Pumpkin Flax Plus Granola
1/2-3/4 cup Nancy's Organic Peach kefir
1 12-ounce can organic peach slices, drained
1 8-ounce carton vanilla bean whole milk yogurt
Agave syrup

Dice bananas and layer alternately with granola in a flat-bottomed, 24-ounce serving bowl, drizzling kefir between layers of bananas and granola. You should have at least two layers but three is possible and preferable with the right bowl. Cover with plastic wrap and allow to set up in the fridge for an hour. Remove plastic wrap and top with peach slices and dabs of vanilla bean yogurt. Drizzle with agave syrup. Serves 2, guiltily.

FIRST QUARTER MOON

MY FIRST DAY BACK FROM BOISE, a day I didn't have to go to campus, the first day with time alone in a week, and all I could do was sleep. I tried to normalize the morning with a trip to Starbucks and the previous week's copies of *The Lewiston Morning Tribune.* The coffee tasted burned and bitter next to the savory batches we'd made at Sean and Susannah's each morning in their expensive drip machine from the Costco bags of Starbucks beans. I was supposed to meet Phil at the Aquatic Center for water aerobics, but I cancelled. It was three p.m. when I called him. I had been asleep three hours, felt disoriented, uncertain of what to do, so I called to say I hadn't made it to the store yet, and if we were going to have anything to eat for dinner, I needed to do the shopping instead. I'd promised him Lasagna al Forno in the wake of all the raving from the Boise faction, with plans to spice it up a bit, hoping to satisfy that hot-tooth he'd developed from sixteen years of living in Texas and still hadn't been able to overcome. I hoped shopping and cooking would be my rescue from what I assumed was post-trip fatigue, and would pull me back into my usual patterns.

At first I thought it was the drive that had so exhausted me. Two hundred-eighty miles in four hours and twenty minutes is pretty fast. As the day wore on, however, it was pretty clear I was fighting an ear infection. I looked at the dollars in my wallet and my shopping list, trying to figure a way to squeeze in a mullein purchase. Any way I looked at it, I was over budget. I decided to forego the convenience of mullein capsules in favor of mullein tea from leaves we'd gathered in the mountains last September and dried ourselves. Mullein is an all-in-one miracle herb. All the world's problems could be solved if we substituted mullein for antibiotics, analgesics, anti-inflammatories, antihistamines, decongestants, and anti-virals. Mullein has also proven to inhibit certain cancers, is an antioxidant, an antifungal, an anti-spasmodic, a diuretic, and a sedative. Basically, if you have a health problem, consume mullein. It will know what to do. It is one of the few herbal medications now solidly backed by research and is widely available and grows wild and abundantly throughout many parts of the world, including North America, Europe, and Asia. You've likely seen it—gray-green fuzzy-leaves low to the ground with yellow flowering stalks several feet tall. In our region of the Inland Northwest, you start seeing it on roadsides at about a thousand feet of elevation. Its recorded use dates back throughout history, particularly in the treatment of asthma and upper respiratory disorders, for which, paradoxically enough, the smoking of the dried leaves is most effective. (No, it doesn't make you high.) As with many plants, some parts are usable by humans and some are toxic. Mullein seeds contain coumarin, the anticoagulant used in "blood thinners" and rat poison, and rotenone, a paralytic Native Americans used to augment fish harvests by paralyzing fish, the ingestion of which has been linked to Parkinson's disease in people. Fish and wildlife agencies use rotenone for wide-spread kills of nuisance fish that compete for habitat with game fish. Ancients also used the stalks for wicks and for dipping in suet to use as torches.

I would never recommend any herb I had not used on myself, and anyone on any other medication should be careful of using mullein. In fact, no one should take my word for any of this at all. Readers should do their own research on the subject and listen to their own instincts. But I would be derelict if I did not broadcast that thrice in two years I have cured ear infections by drinking mullein tea three times a day for ten days. The tea has to be made strong, and it has to be strained well to capture all those fuzzy little hairs than can irritate the throat. But I will swear on a stack of my own journals that mullein tea will cure what ails you. I have found it helps with peri-menopause symptoms, including bloat. I don't recommend using it arbitrarily, and if it is to be used as an antibiotic, strong cups of the tea or forty drops of tincture in water should be taken three to four times a day for ten days and no less—even if symptoms wane, and they will. If capsules are used, a good brand should be chosen, such as Solaray or Nature's Sunshine, and my recommendation (based on my personal experience; the amount likely varies according to weight, so you'd do well to consult someone who is certified to provide dosage advice) is five at a time twice a day for ten days. Before harvesting mullein, do some research about its uses. Go high into the mountains in the autumn before the first freeze. Search along hiking trails to minimize the risk of picking auto-exhaust-fume-contaminated plants. Never pick leaves from mullein with a deformed flower stalk. They should be upright. Bends, curves, or curls in the flower stalk mean the plant is contaminated in some way.

Coincidence or not, I was thinking about writing this section on mullein tea when I ran across an article in a magazine about the many medicinal uses for this wild plant, which included a recipe for a mullein-based detox formula. I've altered it so that it can be used as more of a daily tea for cold and flu season and renamed it "Winter Tonic." Someday when I have the time, I'd like to try making an agave-sweetened sorbet out of it, just for the intriguing flavor combination, although, admittedly, freezing could very well nullify any medicinal properties.

Mullein Cure

1/2 cup dried mullein
1 quart water

For ear and upper respiratory infections, boil mullein in water for 15 minutes. Cool to room temperature. Strain through cheesecloth. Pour 8 ounces into a mug or glass and sweeten with honey. Repeat as necessary to make 3 8-ounce cups a day for ten days.

Winter Tonic

1 tablespoon green tea leaves
1 tablespoon wild cherry bark
1 tablespoon dried mullein leaf
1 tablespoon peppermint leaf

Place dry ingredients in closed jar and shake thoroughly to blend. Spoon into cheesecloth and tie off, then pack into a tea ball. Place ball into mug and cover with boiling water. Steep covered for 15 minutes. Sweeten with agave syrup.

* * *

My friend Jill Nugent had introduced me to mullein back in the fall of 2008 when I was at her house to finish a project we'd been working on. I was at that time also struggling with an ear infection, and she took one look at me, started laying a fire in her wood cooking stove, pulled out a pan, filled it with water from a jug, and dumped a rather large cluster of fresh, sage-green mullein leaves into it. "I knew I picked these for a reason," she said. As she worked, she talked, telling me about mullein's many properties and the story of curing her own pneumonia by drinking a quart of the stuff all at once the winter before. "About five hours later the entire phlegm system came up," she said. "With that one act, I was cured."

Jill was also on my mind that early February day in 2010, when I used mullein leaves to cure yet another ear infection, because it was her healing nature that had also connected her with the people of Haiti, and I'd just received the following email from her, bringing that whole difficult situation in Haiti once again to my mind's forefront. No matter what was going on in our bitsy day-to-day lives, no one, not even the media, could fail to acknowledge the horrifying level of need still in existence among the Haitian people and the fact that they would continue to need help for ages to come:

"The situation on LaGonave: everyone is traumatized, survivors are pouring in from the countryside and food is running out. People in every community are talking,

meeting, walking, and assessing the situation. The Matenwa
Community Learning Center (http://www.matenwaclc.org/)
is working with partner organizations in Port-au-Prince,
such as Beyond Borders (http://www.beyondborders.net/)
and KONPAY (http://www.konpay.org/) on the logistics
of food shipments. KONPAY was told by the UN that
they will not have access to any of the food or medical
aid now pouring in from the big agencies such as
Catholic Relief Services, WorldVision, etc., and they were
encouraged to continue working with the partners they
have to get food and supplies from their own sources.
So they are. They have established connections in the DR
[Dominican Republic] to receive international shipments,
boats from the DR and Cap-Haitian. Grassroots groups
on LaGonave are organizing the distribution system.
Women will come with donkeys to move the food inland
if there is no gas available. Prior to the earthquake the
Courageous Women had been working to build networks
of women's groups in communities remote from the
progressive center in Matenwa, places where people have
little education and don't necessarily even know what an
earthquake is."

Jill's note had me once again comparing my own small existence
to the enormous misery that was Haiti, giving silent prayers of thanks
for the bounty that was my life and the lives of my children.

*   *   *

Phil did his best to listen to my mullein adventures and tales
about what was occurring in Haiti as he prepared a kettle of Hemp
Chili that evening while running back and forth to catch a bit of the
football playoffs. We mused that eating low on the food chain was a
good way to honor those folks who were so suffering. At some point
he stopped to confer on the recipe I was recording as he invented it.
He insisted that such a thing is called simply "beans" down in South
Texas, where "real chili is spiced meat." I at first insisted on keeping

the title, since where I come from, spicy beans with or without out meat are always tagged with the label "chili." Even that stuff they served us in grade school that used spaghetti as a filler.

This was the same guy who decided to call his Sunday vegetarian breakfast offering, "Phil's Mellow Yellow Scramble." (Phil is originally from San Francisco, so perhaps that title is self-explanatory.)

Still, to honor his perspective, I decided to rename the chili. By way of disclaimer, the Muir Glen Fire-Roasted Tomatoes can be expensive, and considering the fates of other people around the world, I am very conscious of how ridiculous this all sounds, but they are the best canned tomatoes I've tried, and I would send a million cases of them to Haiti if I could. Admittedly, I only buy them when they are on sale, and our local grocery liquidator recently had a shipment of them. The celery leaves we dried ourselves.

Spicy Chili Bean Stew

2 cups dried red beans
4 quarts water
1/4 cup sunflower oil
1 large red onion
6 garlic cloves
1 red bell pepper
1/4 cup dried celery leaves, crushed
1 teaspoon dried basil
1 teaspoon fresh ground black pepper
2 teaspoons cumin
2 tablespoons paprika
2 tablespoons chili powder
1/2 teaspoon cayenne
1/2 teaspoon ground coriander
1/4 teaspoon crushed chipotle chili peppers
1 tablespoon agave syrup
2 squares very dark chocolate
2 28-ounce cans Muir Glen Organic Chopped Fire-Roasted
    Tomatoes

1 15-ounce can tomato sauce
Vegetable broth
Sea salt
1/2 cup hulled hemp seed
1/2 cup cheddar cheese, shredded
1/2 cup plain yogurt

Combine beans and 2 quarts of the water in a large soup pot. Bring to a boil. Remove from heat and allow to cool. Drain. Return to pot and add the last 2 quarts of water. Bring to boil. Lower heat and cook uncovered until beans are soft, approximately 2 hours, then set aside. In a separate skillet, sauté onion, garlic, and bell pepper in oil until just starting to soften. Stir in spices, herbs, agave syrup, and chocolate, but not hemp seed. Add mixture to beans along with tomatoes and tomato sauce, using vegetable broth to thin as necessary. Allow to simmer for 30 minutes or so, then sample. Adjust spice and seasoning to taste. Add hemp seed. Do not allow to boil. Simmer on low another 30 minutes. Allow to rest and cool before serving. Top with a bit of shredded cheddar and plain yogurt. Goes great with a handful of organic saltines or crushed tortilla chips.

Phil's Mellow Yellow Scramble

1 tablespoon butter
5 large eggs
2 tablespoons whole milk
1/2 yellow bell pepper, chopped
1 small yellow winter squash (the kind that looks like a
        zucchini), chopped
2 cloves garlic, minced
1/4 cup Tillamook Mexican Blend Shredded Cheese
2 tablespoons shredded Parmesan cheese, plus more for
        topping
Fresh ground black pepper
Tony Chachere's Original Creole Seasoning

Melt butter in skillet. Beat eggs with milk and pour into skillet. Add vegetables and garlic and cook until eggs are no longer runny. Stir in cheeses. Sprinkle with seasonings and continue tossing and stirring until eggs are cooked through. Vegetables will still be slightly firm. Add more seasoning to taste. Top with another sprinkle of Parmesan just before serving.

A few notes on this recipe: Cinnamon-walnut toast made Phil's breakfast a meal to remember. And Oregon's Tillamook Cheese is a more affordable choice than organic. It is pure cheese, and they have built a reputation on only using milk from non-pharmaceutical cows. Lastly, once you get started using Tony Chachere's Original Creole Seasoning, you'll be tempted to use it on everything.

*   *   *

We live in one of the two towns on either side of the confluence of the Snake and Clearwater Rivers where Idaho, Washington, and Oregon share borders. The merged population of Clarkston, Washington, and Lewiston, Idaho, is perhaps fifty thousand. If you go out for beer and The New York Times after the first quarter of the Super Bowl as I did, you will see perhaps thirty vehicles between home and the supermarket—and that includes the ones in the parking lot. You will find plenty of beer—particularly Coors, Pabst, and Budweiser, and in recent years, small-batch microbrews from around the Northwest.

But you will not find *The New York Times*.

Regardless, it was worth the shopping trip since Phil's nachos absolutely required a beer accompaniment. We had discovered Sierra Nevada Brewing Company's Glissade, a golden Northwest pale, and Phil liked Full Sail's LTD Lager. This is one time where I believe it is perfectly permissible to use canned beans, especially from a small-batch, organic company like Oregon's Natural Directions, whose website (http://www.naturaldirections.com/) has a wonderful explanation and argument for buying from small-batch, organic companies. For some reason, refried beans taste better when the beans come from a can.

Phil thinks it's because refried beans are supposed to be made from leftovers. Either way, the great flavor of his three-bean combination surprised me and takes all prizes. He thought so too, apparently, and was inspired enough to give it a rather self-indulgent name.

Phil's Fabulous Three-Bean Nachos

Guacamole:

4 ripe Haas avocados
1 tablespoon mayo
2 tablespoons plain yogurt
2 tablespoons lime juice
Garlic granules
Tony Chachere's Original Creole Seasoning
Fresh ground black pepper

Mash avocado with a fork. Blend with yogurt, mayo, and lime juice until creamy and smooth. Add seasonings to taste. Cover and place in fridge.

Nachos:

1 15-ounce can Natural Directions Kidney Beans
1 15-ounce can Natural Directions Pinto Beans
1 15-ounce can Natural Directions Black Beans
1 fresh jalapeno
2 tablespoons butter
1 teaspoon cumin
Kirkland Organic Tortilla Chips
Kirkland Organic Medium Salsa
2-3 cups Tillamook Vintage White Extra Sharp Cheddar
        Cheese, grated

Preheat the oven to 325 degrees. Cook and mash beans in skillet until well blended. Split jalapeno in half, de-seed at least half, then slice all into 1/4-inch rings. In small skillet, melt butter and stir in cumin. Add sliced jalapeno, cook five minutes, and set aside. Spread a layer of chips on pizza pan, then top with a third of the grated cheese. Spread a layer of half the beans, then half the jalapenos over the chips and cheese. Add another layer of chips, another third of the cheese, the remaining beans, and the remaining jalapenos, then top with rest of the cheese. Bake at 325 degrees for 10 minutes or until cheese is melted. Top with salsa and guacamole.

*   *   *

What a wonderful surprise one morning at the end of February to have Phil say, with his good-bye hug, "Hey! You really are losing weight!" And I was. Hallelujah. Every piece of clothing I put on was just a little bit loose. Well, some things were fairly loose, actually. Loose enough that the way things were going I could see myself tossing them any day. And I did mean to toss them. None of that skinny clothes/fat clothes stuff anymore. These were new habits I planned never to break. And if I did stick with it, I would deserve a new wardrobe. Of all the crosses in life to bear, why mine had to be obesity, I don't know. At age twelve, tired of my family nickname, "Chubby Legs," I saved my babysitting money for a calorie book and went on my first diet. Over my teenage years I took an appetite suppressant called Ayds, many, many times. Ayds looked and tasted just like chocolate caramels, and I'm pretty sure that's exactly what they were, because not once did they suppress my appetite. Just the opposite, in fact. I craved them and bought them to keep on hand in my nightstand for the after-school munchies that descended during that adrenalin-sucking vampire soap *Dark Shadows*.

I guess I understand that I was not made to be a small woman, but I do sometimes wish I did not come from thousands of years of people who had to use their bodies to produce the very same calories their bodies needed to burn to survive. Hundreds of years of Kentucky hill people who sold milk and eggs and stored their annually butchered beeves and hogs in the smokehouse and ground molasses from their own sugarcane by walking a mule around a limestone grindstone. Their lives, beautifully rhythmic and primal, moved with the sun and the moon and the seasons. Both grandpas raised and sold tobacco at the Burley Tobacco barn in Columbia, the county seat and closest town, which was nearly a mile of slate-bottom creek and fifteen miles of dirt road away for my father's father, and about the same number of dirt miles for my mother's family. My body is my physical heritage, handed down by hardscrabble, indigenous people. People whose will and spirit drove them to survive. I use my body to support a pair of eyes and ears and hands and a brain addicted to diction and syntax. It doesn't take much fuel to keep an idle car running. In becoming a vegetarian, I was returning to the ways of my ancestors, the way my body was programmed by generations of people who lived in the same place growing vegetables, fruit, legumes, grains, eggs—and consuming little meat. A Presbyterian cleric who sailed to this country in 1686 and was one of the original Scots allowed to do such; Cherokee great-grandparents who fled the government's forced march to Oklahoma, hid in the Tennessee mountains, and made the babies that became my mother's mother and my father's grandmother; and a slave couple who bore a daughter who fell in love with my father's other grandfather.

I thought of them all as I prepared the house for our friends Ben and Kelsey, who were again scheduled for dinner. On the menu was one of Phil's standards, passed on to him by a former boss in Texas. After much discussion, during which he was unable to remember the name of the type of pasta, I suggested that it sounded like ziti, and devised the title, "South Texas Greek Ziti," at which Phil informed me that Big Bend National Park, where he'd lived previously, is considered to be West Texas, and quite proudly, and that people there definitely wouldn't cotton to being called anything but. The ziti, once we went shopping, turned out to be actually pennoni rigate, a much more bourgeois-sounding name, a smaller noodle than ziti, and less appropriate, I thought, for this thoroughly robust main dish.

Phil's West Texas Greek Company Supper

1/4 cup extra virgin olive oil
12 whole garlic cloves
1 zucchini, cubed
1 yellow winter squash, cubed
1 red bell pepper, cubed
1 red onion, cubed
1 pint whole cherry tomatoes
1 pound pennoni rigate
1/2 cup pine nuts
Fresh basil leaves, torn into bite-sized pieces
Feta cheese

Preheat oven to 350 degrees. Heat oil in oven in glass 9x13 baking dish until oil is very hot. Remove from oven and stir in garlic. Return to oven and bake until you can smell the garlic, about 15 minutes. Add vegetables to oil and garlic and combine well. Bake another 10 minutes or until vegetables just begin to soften. Do not overbake. Meanwhile, cook ziti according to package directions. Brown pine nuts in dry pan over medium heat until toast colored. Place cooked ziti in a serving dish. Pour vegetables on top of ziti. Top with torn basil leaves, then sprinkle with toasted pine nuts and feta. Serve immediately. Keeps well covered in fridge for up to a week.

*   *   *

Phil sent this to the "Letters to the Editor" section of the *Lewiston Morning Tribune*, our local newspaper. It was in reference to the alternating hysteria and paranoia surrounding the reintroduction of wolves to our region. We didn't see what the big deal was. If you have a ranch, you are going to have predators of one sort or another. Cattle and sheep are on everybody's food chain. After watching the film *Two Angry Moms*, about what our children are fed in our public schools across the U.S., Phil couldn't help seeing the irony in a morning news story about some tapeworm in wolves that is deadly to humans. It kills perhaps ten wolves a year in the far north:

> "Dear Editor:
>
> Well, at long last I've up and done it. I've increased my life insurance, and I'm having my house torn down and rebuilt out of brick because I know that any day now the wolves are going to be right outside my door huffing and puffing and trying to blow it down. I'm also going to stop eating because each year there are 76 million illnesses, 325,000 hospitalizations, and 5,000 deaths in the U.S. related to food. Wait! Why am I so concerned about wolves when this is going on with our food? Kinda sounds like I have my priorities mixed up, eh?"

*   *   *

Earlier that February, columnist Kathy Parker had commented on fellow opinion writer Ellen Goodman's retirement, describing the difficulties inherent to producing a regular column day in and day out for weeks, months, and years—in Ellen Goodman's case, decades. The pain and worry and soul-searching involved in keeping awake and alert and absorbing life's minutia and the world so as to capture material enough to keep it fresh, and the grave responsibility such a job brings because the reading public depends on you to be there for them. In not-so-many words, she said it is a cross you have to bear because you believe in the value of the written word and its ability to inspire and improve the lives of everyday folks who still sit down with the newspaper over their morning cups of coffee. Both women became, at that moment, my heroes. Of all the things I've done in my life, I've never done the two things I wanted to do most (and rarely have I confessed these desires to anyone): be a radio announcer and write a syndicated column for newspapers.

As I picture it, the column would be somewhere between Erma Bombeck, Ellen Goodman, Dave Barry, and Garrison Keillor, with liberal doses of Leonard Pitts, Jr. and Molly Ivers. My children, parents, friends, and of course, Phil, would become recurring characters. People would laugh, and people would learn how to enjoy themselves by flowing with life rather than always being in competition with it. I would tell people constantly, "Trust the Force, Luke," because I believe in that. I believe in aligning ourselves with the flow of the natural world and in letting things unfold as they will, hard as that is for me at times in actual practice. I believe all the evil in the world has its beginnings in money—because money is power—and the lust for it, and because power is only craved by the weak. I believe the more and the sooner we move apart from our love affair with it, the better off we all will be.

Some years ago I ran across a little book called, *The Woman Who Lives in the Earth* by Swain Wolfe. The story was set in an earlier time, and the planet was suffering severe drought and heat. All resources, meager as they had been to begin with, were exhausted. The young female protagonist assumed her life was doomed, until she discovered her own relationship with and to the natural world. The book gave language to something I had learned from my father's mother, my Grandma Hazel, and forgotten. Grandma Hazel who taught me the secret of "signs" of looking to the planet itself to guide us in such subjects as when to plant which crops, when to prune, when to can certain fruits and vegetables, when to put up kraut, when to butcher, when to grind cane into molasses. And certain other little things, such as when to know company is coming, when to know someone is lying, when good things are coming, and bad. We don't operate in the world that way in our day, but I was trained to know Grandma Hazel's way exists, and love the world imagined as she and her neighboring "holler" folks imagined it, and find just as much sense in it as I do any other belief system.

Another purpose of my syndicated column, I suppose, might be to explain to the world in a plausible, scientific way why following the cycles of the moon is more logical than plopping down chemical fertilizers, herbicides, and pesticides. (Nobody tells us Americans we are suffering trace element deficiencies because chemical fertilizers cause plant roots to grow too rapidly and too shallowly, preventing them from developing the durability they need to dive deep into the earth in search of sustenance, where they absorb trace elements.) The further I go, the more certain I become that eating a mostly plant-based diet is a quest of the spirit. I believe that when we consume animal flesh we absorb a small amount of the spirit of that animal and its caged-up, fattened-on-the-hoof anxiety. That plants give off a small amount of electromagnetic energy has been well studied and documented. Flesh is formed as the life is lived, so, plant or animal, the life becomes the flesh. (One of the first and best books on plant energy fields and the effects of plant energy is *The Secret Life of Plants*, by Peter Tompkins, and worth reading.) Perhaps it is no wonder that the eradicating power of flower extracts on cancer is one of the most exciting discoveries in medicine so far this century.

When Ben and Kelsey finally came for dinner—weeks after the Buffalo Dilemma—Ben described his one attempt at vegetarianism, explaining that after a few days of not eating meat he began to suffer sweats, nausea, listlessness, even though he had kept track of his protein and felt he was getting enough. Talking with Phil later about Ben's experience, the word withdrawal came to me. How dependent are our twenty-first century bodies on those hormones and antibiotics we've been consuming now for over a generation? Phil and I had been buying, for the most part, organic or local meat from unimpeded, naturally hypertrophied animals not exposed to pharmaceutical intervention, and so far had not experienced anything but wonderment over the changes in ourselves, including a growing sense of peace. Rather than withdrawing from hormones, I'd have to describe it more as finding out what my true spirit is like when I was not sharing its body space with chicken, fish, pig, buffalo, and cow remnants. Perhaps that's why my body grew so large after I left my childhood home and again during my decade-plus-long return to existing as an omnivore—to make room for all those extra dabs of animal soul.

*   *   *

It was bound to happen sooner or later, and later turned out to be the case. The first weekend in March, a convergence of circumstances that led to both of us crashing from low blood sugars: no hemp shake for me on Friday because I'd been engrossed enough in my writing tasks that I'd slipped back into my old habit of not eating until late afternoon, and then settled for a boiled egg and toast instead of making a hemp shake or warming up beans; a Friday night dinner of vegetarian nachos (a very basic cheese and peppers only) that had been delicious but nutritionally meager after an hour of water aerobics; a quick, unexpected overnight visit Friday in the form of Sean and Susannah and the girls on their way through to visit her family in Moscow, which meant a late night and high-energy output; a late breakfast out with them on Saturday at our favorite cafe which was limited to a scone and coffee because the spinach quiche always sells out early.

By the time Sean and his family headed out after breakfast and we'd hit the bank early Saturday afternoon and then started through Costco, I was so weak and nauseated I barely made the return trip to the car, leaving Phil to finish the shopping. Soon enough he came rushing to the rescue with a double box of Mary's Gone Crackers, fabulous organic baked seed crackers made from nothing but rice and seeds. They revived me immediately. The scenario seemed out of whack, until I started the tally I've just relayed here, realizing we hadn't really cooked since Tuesday, and that was Phil's West Texas Greek Company Supper, which was essentially pasta and vegetables, at which point Phil said he thought we were suffering too little protein and too much processed food. We'd had popcorn for dinner Wednesday and take-out vegetarian pizza Thursday night.

Also, my earache had returned. In the end I had wrongfully decided to save our wild-crafted mullein and bought capsules from the health food store. The thought occurred to me: they must contain the death crystals, too. Of course, I don't believe that in those exact terms. But what I do believe is that a capsule full of freeze-dried ground herb is never going to be as potent as what you gather from the wild or grow organically yourself, and that when you make tea, you steep the leaves for quite a while and are bound to ingest more volatile oils than from ground, dehydrated leaves in capsules. Phil reminded me that the last time I'd gotten an ear infection and run out of mullein, I'd had to take dozens of capsules a day, else the symptoms returned. "Besides, we picked that stuff for just this purpose," Phil said, "in case one of us got sick. Go ahead and use it." Of course, spring was nearly here, and we'd soon be able to harvest more.

We made hemp shakes the moment we arrived back home and I drank an entire pint of it in two gulps, followed by two pints of water. Two cups of mullein tea, and I was in good enough shape to invent Baby Lentil Stew and eat a fairly large bowl of it with a handful of Mary's Gone Crackers crumbled in. We realized later, too, that we had learned the blood sugar lesson once already, early on, when I resurrected the recipe for Protein Balls. We simply had to be diligent about keeping wholesome, portable energy sources on hand.

Baby Lentil Stew

2 cups baby brown lentils
4 red potatoes, cubed
4 stalks celery, chopped
1 large white (not yellow) onion, chopped
4 carrots, chopped
4 cloves garlic, chopped
1 8-ounce can tomato paste
2 bay leaves
2 teaspoons thyme
1-2 quarts vegetable broth
2 tablespoons tamari or organic Worcestershire sauce
Fresh ground black pepper
Salt

Rinse lentils and cover in boiling water. Cook over low heat until beginning to soften but leave firm. Drain and add potatoes, celery, onion, carrots, garlic, tomato paste, bay leaves, and thyme. Add enough broth to cover ingredients. Bring to a boil. Cover and simmer until vegetables reach desired firmness. Remove bay leaves. Season with tamari or Worcestershire sauce, black pepper, and salt to taste. Allow to rest uncovered for 15 minutes before serving.

WAXING QUARTER MOON

"Food to a large extent is what holds a society together and eating is closely linked to deep spiritual experiences."

—Peter Farb and George Armelagos in *Consuming Passions: The Anthropology of Eating*

THE IDEALIST IN ME STILL LIVES. Sometimes I have dreams in which we all are different than we are now in waking life. In the dream a way of being has spread through the U.S., an enlightenment set in motion a person at a time, one example spawning the next. A movement so powerful that it quietly, slowly transforms our government processes without anybody noticing. Lobbying falls off because it ceases to be effective. Nobody cares anymore about the big spenders. State and federal political bodies turn themselves to the business of supporting the planet and the everyday lives of regular people, rather than exploiting them, and become more concerned with garden care than health care, because the food we are all eating and the way we are all living has made us too healthy to need health care anyway. The world is, in a word, idyllic. Utopian. In the dream, time has become folkloric and softened. Nobody cares about clocks. People are equally kind, insightful, variously talented, self-sustaining, cooperative, resourceful, peaceful, artful in their ways of doing and being, romantic, fit from spending their days cultivating the nourishment that graces their tables, whether from backyard gardens or community orchards, vineyards, and nut groves. People work hard, celebrate the seasons, and have made a place for technology in education and communication, but it is not visible in day-to-day existence. Each child has been brought to adulthood by wise, loving parents and socialized to the greater whole from birth, such that there is no mental disease, greed, nor love of power, and what few are born damaged are loved and nurtured by the entire community in exchange for being the blessings that they are, for what we all have to learn by caring for them. The fact that human sexuality comes in many shades is not questioned. Nor human skin variations and cultural traditions.

In last night's version of the dream, people were growing tomatoes in pots. The people had decided to no longer purchase food from grocery stores. It was agreed that everyone would grow a small garden, and if for reasons of age or condition they couldn't, they were tasked to place at least a pot of tomatoes in a sunny spot on their front steps—as of course all front steps had sunny spots—so younger folks could come by to water it and to know where their excess vegetables might be welcomed. Everyone traded and bartered for what was otherwise needed. Some people grew wheat; some people grew oats. Each person somehow seemed to know just what he or she needed to grow and share.

Perhaps this version of the dream came from thinking about the best garden spot for tomatoes last night, while standing at the sink as I was making paneer, or Indian homemade cheese, with my own embellishments, of course. But I also knew it was about a last-second decision to visit my parents in Indiana over spring break. It was about wanting for their lives much, more than what I could accomplish for them from a distance. Either way, making paneer gave me a grand excuse to dust off our very cool 1950s glass hand juicer to extract the required lemon juice. When I make it again, I will add salt as well as some olive oil to make it more spreadable, and will use minced garlic instead of granules. As the recipe reads now, it is very mild and the texture more like ricotta, in fact, a very fabulous ricotta, and the cost is about the same as for non-organic ricotta and much more reasonable than for organic ricotta, which I've seen for as much as ten dollars a quart. I likely will freeze it and save it for a lasagna. Still, we happily spread it on Olive Oil and Rosemary Artisan Bread from our local grocery store, broiled it, then dipped it in warmed-over bowls of better-than-the-first-night Baby Lentil Stew.

Garlic-Thyme Farm Cheese

1 gallon organic whole milk
juice from 4 lemons
1 tablespoon thyme
1 teaspoon sea salt
2 teaspoons garlic granules

Bring milk to a boil over medium heat, stirring regularly to keep from scorching. Whisk in lemon juice and remaining ingredients until nickel-sized curds form. Allow to settle and cool slightly. Line strainer with cheesecloth or muslin cheese bag. Pour curds and whey through cheesecloth. Allow to drain for 45 minutes. Bring corners of cheesecloth together and tie closed. Place on flat surface and top with 20-30 pounds of weight or clamp with a vice between two cutting boards. Allow to sit weighted for 3 hours. Store refrigerated for up to one week.

*   *   *

Preparing for a trip home to see Mom and Dad at any time requires a few things, but having it be a sudden decision meant pressure to accomplish a lot quickly. First, beyond the mundane details of airline tickets and itineraries, I had to think about food, not just for the journey but for the visit itself. This has always been the case, since neither of them thinks much about nutrition, which, obviously, is why Dad, in November of 2009, required a quadruple bypass. But then, that is a minor fallacy, since he did manage to keep his arteries clear enough to sustain life in the seventeen years since a massive heart attack shut down his work life. I remember his anger then: "Why didn't they tell us?" he asked, of the deleterious effects of Big Macs and Whoppers.

"It's a conspiracy, Dad," I told him. "It keeps hospitals and pharmacies in business."

He did pretty well, for a while, working out at a gym, riding his bike, bypassing fast food for salad. But age, illness, caring for my disabled mother, a penchant for convenience-store fried potatoes and chicken strips, and a move to a worn, rural side road where riding a bicycle was impossible, all equaled a second myocardial event, hence the bypass surgery and what he now calls having "passed up a beautiful chance to opt out."

This attitude saddened me, and I knew how I would handle it. I would package a container of hemp protein powder and a bag of hemp nut meat. I would scour the local groceries for organic produce, brown rice, yogurt, fruit. I would try, in one short week— once again and as I did every time—to change my parents' dietary habits. It was a daunting task, the results good for about a day, before Dad gave in and bought a quick-stop barbecue sandwich. I knew because that was the first place we went and the first thing he wanted when I'd visited the previous November, just after his release from cardiac rehab. Still, no amount of talking could keep me from trying, no more than no amount of talking would keep him from his quick-stop cuisine—work toward his next beautiful option being his only goal and well underway.

My other challenge was food for the flight. Boiled eggs, celery, and hemp nut meat. Bottled water. And I vowed that would be it. No airport cheese pizza slices. No scones. No who-knows-whose-unwashed hands-and-chemicals-have-been-on-it salads. I tried to think of something else compact to stave hunger, but nothing came. Then Phil showed up with hemp granola bars. He always found a way to save the day.

* * *

Phil's Daily Hemp Shake didn't go over so well with Mom and Dad, despite my best intentions, and despite the new blender I managed to purchase at the Walgreens in Corydon. It wouldn't have gone over well with me either: no kefir, organic or otherwise; no organic yogurt; no organic orange juice; no organic bananas; no sparkling mineral water. Instead, sugar-sweetened Yoplait, mass-produced orange juice that didn't exactly say, "Fresh Squeezed," even, rather "Not from Concentrate," which could mean—what? Made from powdered drink mix? Which is what it reminded me of—that old childhood chemistry experiment, Tang. The final concoction tasted like a grainy supermarket version of the otherwise delicious shakes Phil and I took to work each day. The hemp powder didn't even dissipate. It remained frighteningly suspended. I had planned to introduce Mom and Dad to this new nutrition option, hoping once again to put them both back on the road to health. I was convinced my mother's mental problems were as connected to bad nutrition and environment as Dad's heart disease and diabetes. But much as I tried to reinforce the notion that they need to bypass the cheap, poor-quality canned goods and mass-produced meat they usually bought, my plan was worthless, since they live in an area where folks don't seem to understand the relationship between nutrition, lifestyle, and health, and high-quality food options simply are not available.

The resulting impact is everywhere evident in their region. Hospitals are the central focal points for "health education," cancer, diabetes, and various other support groups, as well as places to get "good jobs," so most people don't notice the fact that they have expanded and proliferated at a rate twice that of the population, along with cancer treatment centers and dialysis centers, which up until recent years were unheard of in any but the most urban areas. (Why is no one noticing the insanely escalating cancer rates, and why is no one thinking about the fact that the diabetes epidemic means that in ten years the amputation rate is going to leave America looking like South Vietnam and that there is a pharmacy on every corner, including Rite Aid and Walgreens in each tiny, rural village, even those with populations under a thousand, speckling the countryside between New Albany and Evansville's one hundred-twenty-or-so mile separation?) Corydon, the population of which is around 2,500, sports not only Walgreens, but a CVS, two mom-and-pops downtown, Walmart's pharmacy, and one inside a locally-owned supermarket. There is one health food store, selling mostly supplements, in Corydon, and one organic food co-op in Paoli, an hour or so from where Mom and Dad's four acres sit. I shop mostly in Corydon at a place called Jaycee's, a Kroger outlet, which has four shelves of packaged organic food items, so I can usually at least make an organic pasta dish, and one shelf of fair quality organic produce. Prices are surprisingly reasonable compared to their commercial counterparts. I point this out to Daddy again and again, but heaven forbid he should pay twenty cents a pound more for organic pasta or tomato sauce or ten cents a pound extra for organic celery, despite the fact that he declares the quality of such food superior every time. And, as I am coming to realize, he will never understand that a penny spent on high-quality food is a dollar saved on "health care." Translation: drug distribution.

All of this was the subject of a long monologue I bestowed on my father on a journey to the big city of New Albany to take back the microwave oven we had purchased the day before from a discount store. It turned out to be not new but refurbished, as was so indicated in microscopic letters on the shipping tag, a label for which we did not even dream we needed to be on the lookout. Long story short, on first try the microwave worked long enough to pop half a bag of death-crystal popcorn, overheated, then died.

"Well, I wouldn't worry about marrying Phil," was Daddy's non-sequitur in response to my little lecture. "He seems like a genuinely nice guy and a good worker. I expect you couldn't do much better."

After which he began to snicker, which built to almost full-blown laughter before it subsided.

"Besides," he said, still chuckling so hard he could barely speak, referencing, I suppose, my two, *ahem,* previous solutions to having wrongly married, "you can always get a divorce."

I interpreted his jab as his way of sidestepping the subject, of avoiding taking responsibility for himself. "If you have knowledge about health, and you don't act on it, it's the same as committing a crime against yourself, Dad," was my way of bringing him back to the subject. I reminded him that I wasn't letting him off the hook, that I wanted him and Mom both to get tested for vitamin D deficiency. Since the last time I'd been to Mom and Dad's, I had gone to a physician's office for help with peri-menopause symptoms. My herbal remedies (Pro-Gest Crème and Estroven) did a good job of relieving hot flashes and moodiness but weren't doing diddly-squat for the fatigue. Blood tests revealed a very severe case of Vitamin D deficiency. The nurse practitioner said it is beginning to be understood as pandemic, particularly in northern climates, such as the one in which I live. The amount of Vitamin D our bodies are able to produce is also affected by changes in the atmosphere and widespread smog and is exacerbated by our increased time spent indoors using computers for work and our use of sunscreen. It is possibly at least partially the root cause of the diabetes, cancer, and heart disease epidemics, all of which are technically inflammatory diseases. People who are low in Vitamin D live with mild, systemic inflammation. She compared it to an automobile being chronically run on only a quart or two of motor oil. Eventually the gaskets heat up, dry out, leak even more oil, and if they are not repaired and the oil is not replaced, sooner or later the engine will seize. She put me on 50,000 units a week. I told Phil that the first doses felt just like that: like oil seeping through and lubricating my joints, muscles, brain, and organ systems. I was immediately more alert and had more energy. All fatigue symptoms disappeared within days, and close friends noticed and commented on my renewed life force much like they did in the first weeks after Phil and I switched to a vegetarian diet. But I would require similar high doses for a year, since I was a mere blood-unit point away from osteomalacia (rickets) and frighteningly close to developing osteoporosis.

Despite my testimony, Mom and Dad both stubbornly refused to be tested for this deficiency, although Dad did agree to a daily 1,000 unit dose which I surreptitiously replaced with 2,000 unit capsules (recommended daily allowances have traditionally been 400 units, but some doctors believe 1,000-2,000 is closer to our modern-day needs). Mom, who went months without leaving the house, insisted she was fine with the 400 units in her daily multi-vitamin.

Symptoms of Vitamin D deficiency mimic many other conditions, which is why it can go undiagnosed: body aches, joint pain, diarrhea, lethargy, excessive sleeping, depression, irregular heartbeat, high blood sugar, high blood pressure, weight gain, food cravings, mood swings, vision changes, inability to concentrate, and bone fracture. Some doctors report that eighty to ninety percent of their patients are proving to be deficient, also thanks to our use of sunscreen and the type of sunrays greenhouse gases prevent from reaching the earth. The deficiency takes years, even decades to produce symptoms for those of us who get at least a bit of exposure to sunlight, so widespread recognition has taken time. The medical community began to notice it after the Taliban moved into Afghanistan and forced females to wear burkas. Within just a few years women were presenting with these symptoms accompanied by softening of bone tissue or osteomalacia.

* * *

Learning that my father was once again considering whether or not to place my mother in a facility where they specialize in caring for people with Alzheimer's was what had my healer self so riled. Mom, who was born severely premature and with deformed legs, and who suffered rheumatoid arthritis and deep depressions most of her life, had been ill for many years with what we had only recently learned could possibly be a very slow form of Alzheimer's. Despite how hard I tried to save her with my diet and nutrition information, and despite my trips back home to buy, cook, and freeze organic meals for both her and my father, it appeared, as much as it pained him, that my father had reached the end of his ability to care for her. Open-heart surgery at the end of 2009 had left him very much weakened and with double vision, and since part of my mother's pathology is hoarding—how do poor people manage to accumulate such a wealth of junk?—leaving little more than a footpath through the rooms of their double-wide, Daddy had fallen more than a dozen times since his operation. For his own health and safety, he was once again thinking he had to let her go.

* * *

A woman I used to know once told me that she had recurring dreams about an asteroid hitting the planet and wreaking widespread and horrific devastation. She was a devoutly religious person and felt certain God was revealing this future truth to her so she might begin preparing her family spiritually and emotionally for such an eventuality. Her dream turned out to be metaphoric, of course, and cataclysm came in the form of her son-in-law committing a crime against a minor and landing himself in prison for seven years, while her daughter bore and raised their son. Once the sentence was served, he was not allowed to live in the same house with his own child for a period of time. When I saw the son-in-law last year at a wedding, the bright, handsome, robust youngster I had last seen in the early 1990s at his own wedding had become dark and hunched into himself. The words "a burned-out star" flashed across my frontal lobe.

Having been raised in a similar religious tradition, thanks to my mother, Armageddon was practically a daily word used to scare us into submission, as was the very expressly described hellfire and damnation. Eventually, I came to believe that the fear of an Armageddon or the end of the world is actually the fear of our own deaths. It makes it possible for me to watch goofy movies like the 1998 blockbuster *Armageddon* without having my sleep subsequently impaired. And what better accompaniment than Phil blanketed on the sofa next to me the night after my return from Indiana, each of us with an Oatmeal-Walnut Burger decked out in lettuce, tomato, and leftover guacamole? Stacked on artisan bakery sourdough rolls, Phil rightfully termed them "Dagwood Burgers." One fist-sized burger was so satisfying, it was all either of us needed for dinner, and this after an hour of intense water aerobics at our local aquatic center.

Besides the fact that you can't buy a copy of *The New York Times*, a list of other oddball details about the area we live in would include the Lewiston Public Library. It may be the only library in the world to share a wall and signage space with a tavern. And a rather sleazy-looking tavern at that—one I had never, nor would ever, check out for myself. But it is the landmark by which most of us provide directions through town: Take 21st Street up the hill and past Rosauer's; take a right into the driveway just past The Wooden Nickel.

Which is exactly the landmark I looked for that following Tuesday, driving in the dark to lead a discussion on Susan Swetnam's lovely collection of personal essays, *Home Mountains*. I have met Susan a few times, although she would not have reason to remember me, but if I meet her again, I would like to tell her just how much her book hit home for me. We are both transplants to this unique region of the world, she in southern Idaho where she teaches in the English Department at Idaho State University. Her words expressed much about how I have felt during the years it took to figure how to survive in a land where people don't coddle, but on the contrary, put great stock in being tough and self-sufficient, while at the same time neighborly and willing to help when times call for it. She reminded me of the years of loneliness I suffered because I did not take the time to meet and know the people around me, never thought to take a meal to a neighbor or enter bread in the county fair or volunteer at the animal shelter. Susan's is a life of giving, learning, teaching, and loving those around her. She is a Brownie leader, a volunteer firefighter, and has a respectable array of research honors and teaching awards.

That night at the library, for some reason, despite the overwhelming generosity of spirit shared between members of the audience and the frankly-spoken and heartwarming compliments directed at me afterwards, by the time I arrived home I had decided that the reason I was not one of the Susan Swetnams of the world, with an armful of published books and plethora of adoring literary fans—in other words, why I am not successful in the way I'd like to be—was somehow Phil's fault. Nothing like a little projection. Of course even a garden mole could figure out that what I was upset about was my parents, my mother. But instead, in an instant, a projectile of deep, deep dismay over the disappointments in my life transformed themselves into a monstrous laser beam of hate pointed directly at Phil. Inexplicable venom burst from this lump between my shoulders and sprayed itself all over this man I planned to marry and claimed to love. He didn't earn it, not in the least, and was deeply pained and flabbergasted by my display. But he stood up for himself, him and his Scorpio stinger, yes they did, and very well, and surprisingly so, given his mild demeanor. What ensued was nothing less than a metaphoric knock-down-drag-out, at times featuring one or both of us screaming, which churned on way into the night until we were both crying and asking each other's forgiveness, both too emotionally exhausted to even sleep, although eventually, at around four-thirty a.m., Phil slowly made his way upstairs to bed.

It was the first of many of these episodes. Whether it was food-related is anybody's guess.

What had started as a discussion about wedding arrangements had ended in a bloody battle that only should have taken place in my own psyche or with a therapist. It was essentially a replay of an old war, my lifelong standoff between what I dreamed my life would be and what it was. Between what was possible for a common Indiana girl according to all those magazine articles and catalog pages and what was not. It is very jealous, that life I did not pursue, the one that would have included me holding UC Berkeley degrees and prancing through my days as a nationally famous and beloved writer of the Barbara Kingsolver ilk or Alice Walker, or even better, a female Ernest Hemingway—without the self-destructive tendencies, without the sexism. In the life I did choose—where I have two stable, brilliant, handsome, talented sons married to stable, brilliant, beautiful, talented women who are intent on making stable, healthy, beautiful homes and stable, healthy, brilliant, beautiful, talented grandchildren for me to spoil and wisely guide—I am simply a middle-aged woman living in the Washington-Idaho outback.

That jealous, left-behind life returned to earth that night in a pompous rage and stayed. Moved right in.

That is the only way I know to explain it. It took me over the way demons in the Bible used to take over people, and perhaps still do.

It was a dark, dark night for both our souls, and Phil and I swore and vowed never to wade into that dank, black territory again.

But we did. Again and again.

What lingered with me otherwise that night, was the way Susan Swetnam wrote about the role food and cooking played in her mental health and helped her cope not only with the big things but also the day-to-day. Comfort found its way to me just before dawn when I finally got the idea that a few carbohydrates might put me to sleep. Comfort in the form of a simple little eight-ounce carton of whole milk lemon yogurt, a chopped banana, and a quarter-cup or so of our artisan bakery's homemade granola. I highly recommend it as a cure for insomnia. Five minutes after I'd finished and brushed my teeth, I was curled under the covers of the downstairs guest room bed, the hand-painted, distressed Pottery Barn farmstead bedframe in which I'd dreamed and fretted and craved sex through almost twenty years of singledom, and to which I am still to this day prone to retreat, always descending quite quickly into the lower realms of sleep.

After the sad and frightening drama left both of us unable to go work the next day, we shouldn't have been surprised by what followed. It was as if the world had decided to remind us of its benevolence and the power of our journey together and about the rightness of our couple-hood. For as long as Phil and I have been living together, we have made a habit of noticing dog ads in the paper. Never until that day, however, had a dog photo made us weep. After we finally found our way to the breakfast table at eleven or so, conciliatory and affectionate with one another, and after I had crawled my way to the car and down to Starbuck's for my morning cuppa, and made my way through the *Lewiston Morning Tribune* to the classifieds section, the first thing my eyes fell upon was the photo of a boxer/Plott's hound mix the Lewis-Clark Animal Shelter was calling, "Ernie."

Why, oh why am I cursed with such a compulsive nature? Emotion, for the ten-thousandth time in my life, overtook me. "Phil," I said, "look."

He did.

And the tears welled for him, too.

He had already begun work on that night's dinner: a shrimp recipe he'd found in the morning paper that interested him as having distinct vegetarian possibilities, so he had started cooking rice.

"We always said we'd know it when we saw it," he said of the dog we'd both, up until that morning, felt neither of us was ready for.

"We're too irresponsible," we had always said. But not in this case. By the time the brown basmati was finished, we were dressed and garbed for a trip to the pound.

How many grown people walk up to a dog cage and start streaming tears? That is exactly what occurred when we walked up to "Ernie's" cage. His boxer/Plott's hound mix manifested as a beautiful, tiger-striped, brindle coat, a boxer body, and the youthful but wise-looking head of a hound, the thing that had stolen our hearts the moment we saw his photo. Both my grandfathers raised coonhounds. Plott's hounds were bred in this country for hunting in the Appalachians and Blue Ridge Mountains. No wonder I thought I was home. "Ernie" seemed just as okay with us as we were with him, so we paid eighty-five dollars and brought him home.

Our only disappointment was that we spent forty dollars on a bag of expensive, brand-name dog food, thinking it to be of superior quality. Turns out it was filled with beet pulp, which is horrible for dogs and an unnecessary fiber filler, as we found once we got home and started researching diets for dogs. Although many people do raise their dogs on a vegetarian diet, we will likely forego it in favor of one of the high-quality meat-based products. Dogs are constructed to be carnivores and foragers. Their modern diets have made them lazy fast-food addicts. It was more than we wanted to think about, trying to guarantee all three of us got enough protein. So, for the moment, at least, Tesla, as we decided to call him, for the great inventor Nikola Tesla, was in dietary limbo as we tried brand after brand of "healthy" dog food.

Phil reinvented the morning newspaper's shrimp recipe as follows, and decided to call it "Tesla's Rice" in honor of the day. The next time he makes it, he'd like to add a few chopped smoky almonds, and I'd agree to the appropriateness of that flavor addition to the dish. I thought a bit of lime zest would further the intrigue, and Phil agreed. The dish stood alone as a meal, and as with many things we have so far cooked, was imminently satisfying, bordering on a comfort food.

Tesla's Rice

> 2 tablespoons sunflower oil
> 2 eggs, beaten
> 1/4 teaspoon salt
> Fresh ground black pepper
> 1 leek, thinly sliced
> 2 carrots, grated
> 1 stalk celery, thinly sliced
> 1 1-inch piece ginger root, peeled and minced
> 1 cup cooked brown basmati rice
> 1 cup cooked white basmati rice
> 1 tablespoon soy sauce

Heat 1 tablespoon oil in a large skillet over high heat. Pour in beaten egg. Season with salt and black pepper. When egg has puffed and cooked through, transfer to plate lined with paper towels. Heat remaining tablespoon oil in skillet over medium heat. Add vegetables and ginger and stir-fry until soft. Add rice and cooked egg, breaking up egg as you toss with vegetables. Add soy sauce and toss again. Serves 2.

* * *

One of the most comforting comfort foods on earth is vegetable noodle soup. My mother made great vats of it until she decided canned soup was superior because of the work it saved her. From then on, it was Campbell's or Ann Page, the A&P brand. Of course, in the 1960s, store-bought soup was not as despicable as it is now. It was real food made from ingredients grown by real hands in real gardens. My brand of vegetable noodle soup evolved from cooking for children and on a very small budget. It is vaguely different each time because the ingredients are unpredictable. For the sake of writing it up in recipe form, I called it, "Icebox Soup," which likely is all the explanation you need. When the forest of leftover noodles and vegetables in the fridge grows dense enough that I have to start shifting things around to unload a trip to the grocer's, you can bet Icebox Soup is about to make an appearance.

Phil and I had yards and yards of frozen leftover egg pasta from a failed Green Hemp Sauce attempt, all of it saturated with butter and olive oil and basil and hemp protein powder and garlic and pine nuts, so much so that I now absolutely recommend liberal doses of all five in any batch of Icebox Soup. Butter and oil, we were discovering, were necessities if we were to remain satiated for any amount of time. Our low-blood sugar dilemma had resolved itself in the wake of my having remembered that a human needs roughly sixty grams or two tablespoons of some kind of fat every day to process certain vitamins, maintain the structure and function of cell membranes, and keep the immune system revved and ready. Saturated fats should be limited to no more than a half-tablespoon per person per day, and since we were using almost no saturated fats, I unabashedly added a bit of actual butter (organic, of course, and of which Costco's Kirkland brand was imminently affordable, especially given the small amounts we were using) to recipes now and again, for the stupendous richness and flavor it lends. All told, we ended up with roughly two gallons of Icebox Soup that next night, ate it for dinner with wedges of bakery-fresh sourdough bread, then lunched the next day on smaller cups of it alongside halves of grilled tomato and cheese sandwiches, also on sourdough, using the mind-bending Vintage White Extra Sharp Cheddar from Oregon's Tillamook Cheese. Dinner was more soup and the other half of that sandwich. I have not a word of description for the soul-mending nature of these meals, either flavor or texture, except to say Rumi would be proud, as every spoonful elicited a satisfied moan from one or both of us, and we felt the benevolent powers of the universe had delivered love to us in the form of Tesla and that soup.

Icebox Soup

2 quarts leftover noodles and/or rice
2 quarts leftover veggies
1 quart leftover beans
1 28-ounce can Muir Glen Organic Fire-Roasted Tomatoes, diced
32 ounces vegetable broth
1/4 cup olive oil
1/4 cup butter
1 tablespoon garlic granules
2 tablespoons tarragon
2 tablespoons basil
1/2 cup dried parsley
1/4 cup Hungarian paprika
1/2 cup hemp seed
1/2 cup pine nuts
1/8 teaspoon crushed chipotle chili peppers
Salt
Tony Chachere's Original Creole Seasoning
Fresh ground black pepper

Combine all ingredients except salt, pepper, and Tony Chachere's Original Creole Seasoning into a very large kettle. Add as much water as needed to thin soup. Bring to boil on high heat, stirring frequently. Immediately lower temperature and simmer on very low heat, covered, stirring occasionally, for 3-4 hours, or use a slow cooker on low for eight hours. Add salt, creole seasoning, and liberal amounts of black pepper just before serving.

NEW MOON

"Dogs love their friends and bite their enemies, quite unlike people, who are incapable of pure love and always have to mix love and hate."

—Sigmund Freud

THAT HOUNDS LOVE TO SLEEP is a thing I'd forgotten. Both sets of Kentucky grandparents had coonhounds, and my mother's stepfather also bred and sold them from time to time. They provided an example of strength and assuredness for my childhood, and I remember the braying, wet noise of them when they came bounding back from a hunt. Nothing stops a coonhound from its prey, certainly not water, especially not the Plott's with their webbed feet. That is the memory I have of them, that and their alerting us to visitors coming long before we could see the whirl of tire dust along those country roads. I bring this up because Tesla had started giving us the evil eye for cooking too loudly and waking him. The click and tap of knives, pans, and spoons annoyed him just enough that he loped into the living room to plop himself on his bed in front of our little gas heat stove.

At first all this sleeping had me concerned the dog was going to be too laid back for us, since we do like to get out and go, and exercise was now a major portion of our day. We finally concluded that perhaps Tesla was still a bit exhausted from his ordeal of life on the streets; being captured by the police after being mauled by some unknown—but from the scars, obviously large—being; then of course, the animal shelter's ritual of vaccines and neutering.

One afternoon a week or so after we got him, however, Phil came in to report having watched Tesla leap twice in mid-air to trampoline himself from deck to yard and yard to deck again. He said he'd never seen a dog leap so far or so high, this after having owned more than a dozen different breeds at various times over the years, and he was certain Tesla's physical prowess was unprecedented. Of course, once the leaping was finished, Tesla was back nuzzling the doorknob and when let in, made his way to the kitchen mat for the nap from which our cooking sounds so rudely—and now predictably—aroused him. Understanding that the boxer half of him was developed to take down boar and bison certainly explained the great leaping action. How far would you have to leap to grab the throat of a fleeing boar or bison? Suffice it to say, Tesla seemed right at home in his current surroundings. He cracked us up with his soft snoring, with his being intent on bestowing us repeat opportunities for petting him, with the way he protected and saved his food, making little stashes of a piece or two to which he'd later return. And, most hilarious, the way he tongued water into his throat in camel-sized gulps, as if recovering from the heat of the desert. At least the sound is what I imagined a camel refueling from a trek in the hot sand might make.

The meal we were busy with that night was Oatmeal-Walnut Loaf, which took advantage of the leftover half of the mix we used for burgers previously, and a variation of "Tesla's Rice" Phil wittily decided to call, "Eggless in Clarkston," in response to my asking whether the dish was once again going to include egg, which seemed like a bit much considering the rich nature of Oatmeal-Walnut Loaf. As usual, dinner was satisfying and wholesome, and we finished well-nourished and energized enough to engage in a game of Triple Yahtzee, the sound of which interested Tesla such that he stood nose-to-corner with our breakfast table, which is tall like a tavern table, watching and watching and cocking his head to yet one more peculiarity in his new surroundings.

Oatmeal-Walnut Loaf

1/2 recipe Oatmeal-Walnut Burger
1/2 cup leftover beans, any kind, mashed
1/4 cup hemp seed
1/4 cup ketchup

Preheat oven to 325 degrees. Mix first three ingredients very well and place in loaf pan. Decorate with ketchup. Place a few tablespoons water around edges of pan. Cover with foil. Bake for 40 minutes, then remove foil and allow to bake another 10 or so minutes, or until edges of loaf are golden. Serves 4.

Eggless in Clarkston

1 tablespoon olive oil
3 garlic cloves, finely chopped
1 stalk celery, thinly sliced
1/3 red bell pepper, chopped
1/2 leek, thinly sliced
1 1-inch piece ginger root, peeled and minced
1 cup cooked brown basmati rice
1 cup cooked white basmati rice
1 tablespoon tamari sauce
Crushed chipotle chili pepper
White pepper

Heat oil, garlic, and celery over medium-high heat until celery just starts to soften. Add bell pepper, leek, and ginger. Stir fry until bell pepper is tender but still slightly crisp. Add rice and tamari. Season with chili pepper and white pepper to taste. Serves 4.

* * *

Finally we managed to get ourselves to our favorite bakery/cafe in time for the spinach quiche. Saturday mornings were busy there, and unless you arrived before nine a.m., a vegetarian wasn't likely to find much to eat beyond sweets. We used to, as omnivores, try to get there before all the savory galettes were gone—little rustic tarts filled with potato, ham, green pepper, egg, and cheese. The crust was flaky, layered, buttery, and astonishing—filled with, I'm sure, half a day's supply of fat and sodium, but they fueled us until dinnertime, so we figured it was a fair trade. The only vegetarian galettes the café made were fruited and sugary; likewise their scones now seemed far too sweet. So we were down to spinach quiche, and that particular Saturday was the first time since New Year's we'd made it in time to enjoy some. Funny. About four bites in, we both said the same thing, almost simultaneously, "You know, we could do this at home." But the main point of the outing was Tesla. We wanted to see how he would behave if left sitting in the pickup, since he had shown a tendency to chew things when we left the house with him locked in the utility room. If his first stay alone was any indication, he was going to be a great boon to the recycling industry, having shredded most of the stack of cardboard waiting to be carted away, the clean-up of which was pretty damned annoying. Still, we tried to make light of it, chalk it up to him exploring his new surroundings. We half expected to return to find the steering wheel gnawed or the leather gearshift knob shredded, since he'd also chewed up a sofa pillow just the day before. I snuck peeks at him twice under the guise of showing him off to the café staff, and both times he was merely seated, taking in the world with that infinitely curious, ears-up, heart-melting pose of his.

Phil and I both have the habit of picking up feathers when we find them. Both our vehicles have a stash of them. In mountain mythology and Native American teachings, the Creator delivers either medicine, protection, or blessings in the form of feathers, so if you see one you'd best pick it up and save it, else you won't have whatever help/mojo you're going to need when you need it. All we found altered upon our return to the truck were two wet feathers. On our way home, Tesla only had to be told "No!" once, when he got just a little too close to our bags of bread (one walnut-raisin and one sourdough) and the clamshell container holding our single slice of raspberry-white-chocolate-mocha moussecake, which is a confluence of mocha mousse and cheesecake topped with a layer of white chocolate ganache and fresh raspberries and, like all this particular bakery's desserts, is nirvana on a fork.

Having just paid to print and mail our "Save the Date" cards for our May wedding, this slice of moussecake was to serve to celebrate the occasion and, as we decided to declare it, a very belated Valentine's Day, even though I did buy us a bar of chocolate-covered marzipan on February 14th. Phil was impassionate about such holidays, and I have come to prefer the way he surprises me throughout the year with flowers and small gifts, rather than responding to the forced expectations Valentine's Day generates. My brother Jacob (yes, I have a son Jacob and a brother Jacob, and to confuse things further, Phil has a brother Jacob, too) calls it, "Get It Right Day." What a ridiculous occasion: Phil is expected to buy me something, and I am expected to believe his purchase is evidence of his love. Much better that, on any other day, I should come home tired from work to a lovely bouquet or that I should, on a whim in the middle of winter, stop at the co-op and pick up for him organic posies grown in local hothouses. Or that he should stop at our local hometown pharmacy and gift shop on the way home and buy me a card, for no reason at all. Or that we should decide in mid-March to buy moussecake.

Phil's real gift came to me the next day, when he was to take Tesla with him to his National Park Service office, ten miles east of us in Spalding, Idaho, trying to catch up before his deadline on all the purchase and project requests to be funded by American Reinvestment and Recovery Act monies, and I was to be home alone for the first time in ten days, the house quiet and my time free.

I planned to forget for a while what it was like to have a dog, as soon as I'd cleaned the mess in the utility room, cleared it of all things destroyable, mopped the kitchen floors, vacuumed the rugs, and run out to purchase a greater array of chew toys, hoping what seemed to be Tesla's one anxiety would eventually exhaust itself. It was taking more energy than either of us had imagined, and I, especially, had no patience for this dog's habit of shredding things. "You have no tolerance," Phil had said to me the night before, and he was right. I didn't.

I had an email from my friend and fellow Kentucky native, author Ed McClanahan, after he'd looked up Plott's Hounds, found them beautiful, and claimed that hounds have always been his favorite dogs. He wrote: "I'm reminded of this old song—'Every time I go to town, the boys all kick my dog around. Makes no difference that he's just a hound, they gotta quit kickin' my dog around!'" Of course, there was no "just" in our description of Tesla. We knew he was more than any mere hound, even with his mildly annoying habits. And after what turned out to be a very stress-free afternoon at his office with Tesla, Phil speculated that perhaps we soon were going to see re-emerging the bright, gentlemanly dog we had witnessed on that first day.

We were quite amused when at nine p.m. or so that night, Tesla clearly had decided it was time for bed. He paced and paced the living room, even after being let out to "go potty," kept pasting his nose to the glass panes of the French doors between the living room and the upstairs foyer, and did not cease until we opened the doors and carried his bed up to our bedroom. He galloped up and down, loud as a horse, until I finally gave in, brushed my teeth, and climbed the stairs myself. He did not stop pacing, however, as was heralded by the tinkling of a pair of brand new tags, until Phil arrived ten or so minutes later. "How cute," we said. "He's herding us."

We were not so amused when, during the night, he vomited partially digested grass shoots and daffodils one puddle apiece on each of our five-hundred-dollar Egyptian rugs.

* * *

I hoped I was not becoming so accustomed to Phil's Sunday breakfasts as to take them for granted, because certainly, once again, he had outdone himself with his Pepper-Onion-Garlic-Cheese Omelet. Funny how the tiniest change of ingredients can alter a recipe entirely.

Thanks to this phenomenon, the Three-Bean Cheesy Spoonbread I modified from an old-time, down-home dish the night before was also a flavorful, nourishing success when warmed over for Sunday dinner. It was the sort of meal that needed to rest before serving, but by the time I had finished the charge to create indestructible puppy space on Saturday afternoon, dinner was very late, and we were too starved to wait. Sunday was no less frenetic given the fact that Tesla, who had apparently grown more comfortable with his surroundings overnight, had started punctuating his discontent. This he exhibited by defecating while closed up in the newly puppy-proofed utility room that morning as we went for coffee (What? No cardboard to chew? Well, I might as well just shit!). He also let us know that he did not like being closed in the rather large dog run that sat unused and overgrown at the back of our property. Despite the fact that Phil spent a good part of Monday, a personal leave day taken just for this purpose, de-ivy-ing the tightly-constructed, cozy little dog house inside it and adding two feet of height to the fence, we suspected Tesla howled the entire time we were gone to water aerobics in the afternoon, since he did so for the minutes we waited in the driveway trying to decide if we should leave (we left), and was still howling hoarsely when we returned. This fact became very obvious as soon as we turned the corner onto our street—we could hear his wail even with the car windows up. Saddened by this new behavior (we were now haunted by the words of the animal shelter volunteer—"Nobody's taken him because of his barking"—and the phone call Saturday from a Shelter worker who was amazed that barking—read "howling"—hadn't been a problem), and weary from two days of this kind of problem solving, we decided our last resort was to try leaving Tesla loose in the yard and pray he didn't find a way to get out. The plan for Tuesday was to stop by the police department to leave Phil's office phone number, just in case some neighbor called in to complain. (We have at least one neighbor who works shifts and sometimes sleeps during the day). We determined otherwise to go about our business and pray for the best.

Phil's Pepper-Onion-Garlic-Cheese Omelet

    2 tablespoons butter
    1/2 red bell pepper, chopped
    1/4 white onion (not yellow), finely chopped
    2 cloves garlic, minced
    5 eggs, slightly beaten
    2 tablespoons whole milk
    1/3 cup grated Tillamook Vintage White Extra Sharp
            Cheddar Cheese

Sauté vegetables and garlic in butter in omelet pan over medium heat until onion is transparent. Remove from pan and set aside. Beat eggs with milk. Pour into pan. Cook over medium heat until egg is set. Sprinkle with cheese and vegetables on one half. Fold plain half over vegetable half. When cheese is melted, flip omelet. Serve immediately with sourdough toast and strawberry-rhubarb jam.

Three-Bean Cheesy Spoonbread

Beans:

1 cup black beans
1 cup pinto beans
1 cup kidney beans
6 quarts water
1 tablespoon yellow mustard
1 tablespoon garlic granules
2 teaspoons rosemary, crushed
1 teaspoon cardamom
Crushed dried chipotle chilis
Salt to taste
Fresh ground black pepper

Place beans in a large soup pot. Cover with 3 quarts of the water and bring to a boil. Remove from heat and allow to cool. Drain. Return to pot and cover with remaining water. Cook on low heat for 1-2 hours, until just starting to soften, making sure there is plenty of water to form a juice. Add herbs and seasoning. Simmer on very low heat, covered, for 2-3 hours. Allow to cool while baking spoonbread.

Spoonbread:

2 cups unbleached flour
1 cup oat flour
1/2 cup cornmeal
1 teaspoon baking powder
1/2 teaspoon salt
1/4 cup plus 2 tablespoons sunflower oil
1 egg, slightly beaten
1 tablespoon agave syrup
1 cup milk
1/2 cup grated Tillamook Vintage White Extra Sharp
        Cheddar Cheese
1/2 cup melted butter

Stir together flours, cornmeal, baking powder, and salt. Make a well and add 1/4 cup oil, egg, agave, milk, cheese, and the melted butter. Stir, adding water until a thick batter forms. Oil cast iron skillet with 2 tablespoons sunflower oil. Pour batter in skillet. Cook covered, over very low heat on stovetop until bread is firm, about forty-five minutes. Place in oven on low broil until golden brown. Allow to set up until completely cool, about two hours or overnight.

Rewarm beans and spoonbread. Use a large serving spoon to lift portions of spoonbread into bowls and ladle on beans. Top with ketchup and hot sauce as desired. Makes 8 hearty portions.

* * *

We all know these people: the sort who, when they visit other people, under the premises of taking a powder, silently open and peer into the bathroom medicine cabinet looking for secrets; the kind who, if they find their host's chocolate stash, will eat it all, quiet square by quiet square, in the middle of the night, thinking each time no one will notice if they take just one; the kind who, despite all the love and devotion and efforts and good money spent on their behalf, will leap the fence in the middle of the afternoon, mere hours before their owners are due home, and land themselves back in jail, no different than your average junkie. And so evolved the scene at our little breakfast table Wednesday morning after an evening of pondering, pondering, pondering, chewing and toying and turning the situation six ways from Sunday, whereby we asked ourselves the question, "Do we want him back? Is Tesla merely having separation anxiety fueled by trauma and puppydom or is he bipolar? Schizophrenic? A con artist?" And the other stupid questions: "Why didn't the animal shelter call Phil at work so he could fetch Tesla on the spot instead of filling our answering machine with long, curly-cued pleas tinted with consternation? And why didn't the police, considering I'd purposefully stopped in the morning before, left Phil's office phone number, and explained the situation and how Phil's office is a mere twenty minutes away and how much we'd prefer he drive in and retrieve Tesla rather than re-expose our dog to the atmosphere of the pound? But the worst, most horrible question was, what if we don't really want a dog? What if we got him, you know, to ignore the deeper reasons behind that big fight?

That, and what was I to do with the tears of a grown man whose ex-wife somehow managed custody of a dozen rescue dogs with whose care and nurturing he'd been charged throughout their ten-year marriage? "It took me more than an hour every night after work, just to feed them all," he told me, sharing again the story, "and that doesn't count having to walk them all every day." I'd seen photos and a video of those animals, and you would never know they had been strays such was their health, exuberance, and vibrancy. Had he decided to face his fear of heartbreak only to have it come to this?

"But think," I told him as we were getting ready for bed, "how many times after I moved in did I try to run? What if Tesla is so used to fending on his own he is afraid of what it feels like to be secure?" What if, the stillest part of myself whispered—the self that didn't want to own up to it—Tesla is, as my brother Jacob insists, a projection of me? Whatever the answers to those questions were, the situation certainly wasn't hurt by a meal of Sweet Lentil Polou, which I adapted from a *Laurel's Kitchen* recipe. I used baby brown lentils, but any variety would work just as well. Dried raisins, apples, or cranberries in place of the currents also work, as do walnuts or almonds in place of the pine nuts.

Sweet Lentil Polou

> 1 tablespoon extra-virgin olive oil
> 1 small red onion, finely chopped
> 1 bay leaf
> 1 cup cooked brown basmati rice
> 1 tablespoon tomato paste
> 3 cups vegetable broth
> 1/4 teaspoon cinnamon
> pinch cardamom

1 cup baby brown lentils
1/2 teaspoon salt
1/4 teaspoon white pepper
1/2 cup dried currants
1/2 cup pine nuts

Preheat oven to 325 degrees. Sauté onion and bay leaf in olive oil over medium heat until onion is soft. Discard bay leaf. Add rice and stir until hot throughout. In a small bowl, mix tomato paste, broth, and spice. Add mixture to rice along with the lentils. Bring to a boil, cover, and simmer on very low heat for 30 minutes. Stir in seasoning, fruit, and nuts. Pour mixture into covered casserole. Add very hot (not boiling) water as necessary to create a thick soup. Cover and bake 20-30 minutes. Serve with salad or vegetable raita. Serves four liberally.

*   *   *

If it weren't for Phil's Daily Hemp Shake, I would have keeled over from lack of blood sugar the next day, since the time consumed by retrieving Tesla left none for eating, not to mention the energy drain of having spent a night and day in the emotional black hole of such decision-making. Agreeing to remain Tesla's "people" required painful examination of our motives and several trips back and forth between the animal shelter and the Lewis Clark Valley's pet supply retailers. In the end, one thing mattered: we had fallen in love with this animal because we each felt such kinship with him. Phil, with his Russian-Swedish-Danish-Latino blood, and I, with my Scottish-Cherokee-African heritage, know what it is to be derived from polar genetics.

Even if we had found Richard B. Woodward's article "Great Plot! The Toughest Dog on the Planet Makes its Debut at Westminster" earlier, we doubt it would have changed our minds. Plott's hounds, it turned out, have very close memories of their wolf beginnings. They miss curling up safe and sound in their dens. So it was that we were one hundred and fifteen dollars poorer, thanks to the purchase of a large dog crate, a water bottle that looked as if it were designed for an overgrown hamster, and a fake-granite food bowl, both of which attached to the inside of the crate door. A pile of old throw rugs and a jerky treat thrown to the back of the crate was all it took. Tesla was home, and so were we, and Phil made Tesla's Rice to mark the day. What follows is excerpted from the February, 2008, online edition of *Slate Magazine*:

"... the Plott hound has been the state dog of North Carolina since 1988 and a common sight for more than a century in eastern Tennessee, where, by one owner's estimate, 'about every third dog tied up back of someone's house is a Plott.' Unless you've hunted black bear or wild boar, or you've spent a lot of time in the Smoky Mountains, you've probably never heard of, much less encountered, a Plott hound.

... Outdoorsmen from as far away as Africa and Japan hold the Plott in near-mystical esteem as the world's toughest dog. Bred to track, run down, tree, and grapple with a baying 500-pound bear eight times its size, it is often overmatched but rarely chastened by that fact. Inspect the coat of one that has worked in the woods for a year or more, and you will likely find slash marks from a bear's claws or a hog's tusks. Plotts routinely will stay on game, alone or in packs, for days at a time. Willing to sacrifice themselves before they'll run from a showdown, they are the ninja warriors of dogdom. By comparison, the beagle is a layabout, and the pit bull a pansy.

... The cult of the dog is best sampled in back issues of the annuals published by the National Plott Hound Association and the American Plott Association. Along with photos of deceased bear, boar, mountain lion, and raccoon draped over pickup trucks, the pages are filled with moving encomia to the mettle of old Plotts, living and dead. Owners will often boast about their dogs when they've 'pulled hair' (bitten a bear). Breeders may hyperbolize the tracking nose of a beloved stud ('able to cold trail and jump a bear, after the track has been boohooed, foot raced and gave up on') or relate harrowing tales of a season just past. ('I had four dogs injured before the bear was killed. Susie, Betsy, and Chuta ... were all bitten badly. The bear had Chuta's whole head in its mouth but she survived.') "

*   *   *

On an afternoon later in April, one of my students came to me with tears in his eyes. He was the one who had revealed during a break-the-ice activity early in the semester that he had made the switch to organic foods and had begun meditating on a daily basis. A graduating senior in his final semester of college, he was worried about his grades in my professional writing class; he was struggling, having difficulty focusing on schoolwork. His father was recently diagnosed with cancer; his grandfather had passed in January; and his relationship of five years had dissolved at the same time. Life had changed him, he said. No longer did he want a Rolex and to own his own jet—a dream that pleased his father, an uneducated man of self-made wealth. When this young man revealed his change of heart to his father, that he wanted to turn his business degree into a PhD, that he wanted to become a university professor to "teach others going into business to look at business and finance in this new, more human way," his father told him he was daft. "I find myself trying to teach my father and my former girlfriend what I see," the student said. "I want to help them. Now I see that life is not about money. But Dad thinks it's the stress making me feel this way, and my ex won't have anything to do with me. They don't believe me when I tell them I've changed. They think I'm going through a phase."

"You've evolved," I told him. "You've passed into a new stage of development and you can't let anybody hold you back. Sometimes in life you make hard choices. You may find yourself losing your supporters. That's life's challenge. Hold on and keep going. Eventually your father will find his way to where you are, and he will do it because he loves you and wants to know you. You will become the embodiment of what he was unable to be."

By the time I had spoken those sentences, the student was no longer blinking back tears. I could see certainty rising in him. He felt in his body that what I had said was true, and said as much. Despite feeling a bit like a soap-opera Yoda, I heard myself, too, talking to myself about Tesla. I heard myself saying, "Hold on and keep going."

After spending the entire day dreading the trip home, putting off the drive as long as feasible, white-knuckling the steering wheel against whatever drama awaited, I was irritated to the core two hours later at being the first to arrive at our lovely Clarkston home. Was Tesla dead in the crate? Or, conjuring a scene an acquaintance had shared with me about her dog-ownership experiences after I'd relayed the story of Tesla—was he toothless and bloody from having chewed his way out of its metal grate door?

But no. He only acted like he wished he were dead, rolling and groveling like a junior clerk. Was I truly so unprepared for him to have scraped back a pair of throw rugs, defecated in the corner of his crate, curled himself pill-bug fashion and waited out a six-hour stay in his "den," just like everyone said he would if the carrier were too big?

Still, we'd survived another day. Another twenty-five bucks for a pillow large enough to take up space in the back of the crate, along with a few bricks meant to decrease the amount of comfortable space, which constituted the next goal for Tesla's "cognitive therapy." After he'd managed another pair of pole vaults over the fence (he figured how to leap onto the brick of a flower bed and pounce against the house, leveraging enough momentum to get over the top of our chest-high fence), now even his toileting was supervised. But, and I hated to say it, lest I jinx it, he was showing signs of "getting it," as I knew my student's father eventually would, too.

Phil took Tesla on a very long walk after work, and I am proud to announce we went out on our own for a while too—left Tesla alone in the utility room and returned an hour later to find it absolutely intact. We made a virtual party of praising his behavior, bestowed on him the holy and almighty jerky treat, after which he proudly lay in his favorite spot, on top of his big, round doggy bed in front of the fire, leaving us to a rousing game of Triple Yahtzee and a dinner of leftover Three-Bean Cheesy Spoonbread, albeit without the spoonbread. A tablespoon of ketchup and a few slices of fresh Sage Bakery Sourdough turned those lowly bean leftovers into a feast. Dessert was easy and instantaneous. A spoonful of strawberry-rhubarb jam we'd bought at the Farmer's Market the summer prior lavished on that toasted sourdough.

*   *   *

I remembered a poster I had seen once. It showed young children how to make food choices based on color, and one of the things it emphasized is to eat more greens and yellows than anything else. What a memory trick. Food as paint. Why it had not occurred to me to consider cooking as way of creating with color before, I do not know. Phil, charged with making a salad, asked me if I intended to use the co-op vegetables I'd purchased the day before for anything in particular. "No," I said, "I shopped by intuition, not with a list. You know, like buying a bunch of colors of paint and then going home to paint a picture you didn't know you wanted to paint." As someone who has long toyed with the idea of going to art school, I am prone to analogies involving paint. At that moment, I noted the lovely rustic color of the beans I was cooking and decided to consider them as assemblage art. I had already unabashedly dropped in a two-tablespoon cube of butter. It melted into a pool of the exact same shade of butter pale it had always been, only its physicality transformed. I felt I wanted to add more oregano (our own fragrant hot Italian oregano we grew last summer and dried ourselves) and wondered what effect it would have if I crumbled more on the surface and left its spruce-greenness lying there, topping it with the black and gray of cracked pepper, and without stirring it, so that my skillet of kidney beans would appear as a cross-section of earth and rock, those added flavors slowly filtering to the bottom.

Which is exactly the point I walked over to the breakfast table to type feverishly about the experience into my laptop.

And also the exact moment Phil walked over to the stove with one of our new bamboo cooking spoons and started stirring my beans. I actually screamed. He couldn't have felt worse, of course, and I couldn't explain what was wrong lest I appear too daft, so I was doubly glad when he accepted my apology and my meager reference to an "experiment that didn't matter" and the endeavor turned into one of our most satisfying and delicious meals yet. What started out as slow-cooker kidney beans—a great idea, by the way, we finally realized, to have some basis to begin a meal after a day's work—wound up as what could only be described as a taco salad. We decided that when we make it again, we will add chopped avocado and some grated Monterey Jack cheese. Also, we have recently discovered Costco's Kirkland Signature Organic Medium Salsa and highly recommend it. It is as good of a store-bought salsa either of us have tasted in a while. And their organic tortilla chips are top-notch as well. And I promise that screaming will be the last thing on your mind, nor will you miss the meat.

Mighty Fine Taco Salad

2 cups dried kidney beans
2 quarts filtered water
1 cup uncooked basmati rice
1-1/2 cups water
2 tablespoons sunflower oil
1/2 large white onion, chopped
1 heaping tablespoon hot Italian oregano
2 tablespoons butter
Fresh ground black pepper
1 head romaine lettuce, chopped
2 tomatoes, diced
1 leek, chopped
1 head red cabbage, chopped
1 cup grated sharp cheddar cheese
1 avocado, chopped
Cayenne pepper to taste
Medium salsa
Tortilla chips

Soak beans overnight and drain. Cook on low in a slow cooker in 2 quarts filtered water for 9 hours. In a medium pan, soak basmati in 1-1/2 cups water for 20 minutes. Place over medium heat and bring to a boil. Cook over very low heat, covered, for 20 minutes. Remove from heat and set aside, covered, until ready to use. In a large skillet, sauté onion in oil until caramelized. Add cooked beans and half the oregano and stir. Cook beans, partially covered and at a hard simmer, until half the juice is boiled off. Add butter. Top with the remaining oregano and lots of fresh ground black pepper. Simmer for 15 more minutes, cover completely, and turn off heat. Meanwhile, make a tossed salad of chopped romaine, tomato, leek, and red cabbage. You will need 2 cups of salad per serving. Arrange salad on a dinner plate and top with cooked basmati. Sprinkle with cheese and chopped avocado. Spoon beans over rice. Sprinkle with a few dashes of cayenne, then top with salsa and crumbled tortilla chips. Makes enough beans and rice for 4 generous servings.

* * *

Phil has a way of taking the most basic ingredients and rearranging them to create something lovely and satisfying. I met him at a time in my life when I was very unhealthy from working and worrying too much and not taking sufficient care of myself. Dinner in those days was often a can of tuna. Our very first date featured one of Phil's home-cooked meals of pork tenderloin, potatoes rinsed of their excess starch, then cooked and mashed with butter, and steamed veggies. All very basic, but all wonderfully seasoned with Tony Chachere's Original Creole Seasoning, of which we are both now ardent fans. It adds a nice bit of heat and a kind of spice I have not found in any other seasoning. It is the one thing we buy that is not organic, but I love that it comes from a small company based in Opelousas, Louisiana, still operated by the grandson of its inventor, Tony Chachere, who published a creole cookbook featuring the now famous seasoning, eventually opening his tiny spice company in 1972.

One night later in April, Phil came up with this simple but lovely recipe we finally decided to call Garden Lentil Soup. It stood on its own and was the perfect end to a day that started with a long morning walk, included Phil nailing up a temporary "hillbilly fence" atop the permanent fence to obscure Tesla's now infamous escape route, and leaving Tesla crated for three hours without incident while we attended "The World's Largest Yard Sale" at the Nez Perce County Fairgrounds in Lewiston. I bought a Remington Typewriter from a former University of Idaho administrator for twelve dollars. She said she used it to get herself through her undergraduate degree and that it had been covered and stored, completely unused, in the decades since. We wanted to have it serviced, hopefully find a new ribbon, and feature it in our wedding as a place for people to type small stories and poems. Phil made a miraculous buy of a set of golf clubs in a beautifully kept vintage leather bag with a pull-cart for three dollars. He entertained himself and Tesla for quite a while slamming golf balls into the shrubs in the late afternoon. The depths of our backyard still harbors a single, unrecovered ball.

Garden Lentil Soup

1 cup French green lentils
1/2 cup baby brown lentils
1 cup diced white onion
5 cloves garlic, minced
4 quarts water
3 carrots, cut into 1/4-inch slices
2 cups chopped bok choy
Tony Chachere's Original Creole Seasoning
Fresh ground black pepper
Salt

Add all ingredients but carrots, bok choy, and seasonings. Bring to full boil. Simmer for 1 hour or until lentils are soft. Add carrots. Cook 10 minutes or until carrots are partially soft. Add bok choy and simmer 2-3 minutes. Season to taste. Makes 6 generous servings.

* * *

I was reading *Imagining Australia: Literature and Culture in the New, New World*, a collection of scholarly essays on Australian literature edited by Judith Ryan and Chris Wallace-Crabbe and published by Harvard University Press. Not many people read these sorts of essays, but I was hoping to propose a course in Australian literature the next year, and such books were required preparation. Australia has long held my fascination, as it does for many Americans. I had been for several years working on a novel set partially in a 1960s Western Australia, and Phil and I both had the uncanny ability to rent videos, only to discover once we had the film home that it was set in Australia. As a consequence, I have viewed hundreds of movies about Australians, have read dozens of Australian memoirs and nonfiction accounts of Australian history and its people.

One essay in the *Imagining Australia* collection featured a quote from prize-winning Australian author Jacob Malouf, who ended a famous lecture series on the making of Australian consciousness and culture with the following sentence: "...acting imaginatively in the spirit of lightness... is the way to wholeness; and wholeness, haleness, as the roots of our language tell us, is health."

My own heritage brings with it a bit of blackness known as "Appalachian fatalism." It is a mindset, an attitude, which comes from living in declivities in the earth ("hollers") where the sun is slow to reach each morning and quick to depart each afternoon. In the West we call this mindset, "canyon mentality." It is the effect of low sunlight on the body resulting in low serotonin levels and translates over a period of generations to a sense of expecting the worst, expecting failure and disappointment. That and a long history of being culturally ignored while enduring media jokes and ridicule. (*How can you tell a hillbilly's been to town? Jealous sister.*)

I have days when remnants of that fatalism overtakes me. Days when there is nothing I can do but go to sleep to have my dreams explain things to me. It feels as if I have to sleep, the way a narcoleptic must feel, and I have to sleep now because I need to dream whatever dream is gnawing at me. Whether it was fatalism or exhaustion, I could find no use for myself that next to the last weekend in April other than the couch and *Imagining Australia*. Phil drove out to his office and took Tesla with him. Dinner was to be leftovers. Self-pity sleazed its way in; self-loathing knocked. I toyed with the notion that there was no good use in the entire world for me.

And then Malouf's statement forced me to look up at the blue-sky-happy day outside and ask myself why I wasn't out in it. It's the last thought I remember. Awakened hours later by Phil's phone call saying he was on his way home, I bounded from the couch rejuvenated, buoyant. For nights I had been dreaming about my ex-husband having an affair and marrying another, a thing he actually did. These I tried to categorize as anxiety dreams. Anxiety over committing to a new life with Phil. A new normal. But I worried they were predictions. Another inherited characteristic: my mother always feared the possibility that my father would have an affair. I pushed it from me. Phil was loyal. Phil was not my ex-husband.

The sleep had led me to one other thing. Downtime may be necessary, dreamtime may be necessary, but I much preferred "acting imaginatively in the spirit of lightness." Australian aboriginals believe dreaming is our one actuality, our truest form of being. For them, only the dreamtime matters. Dreamtime is living. Awaketime is sleeping. They reproduce the messages of the dreamtime to assist with deciphering images found in awaketime. In our world we call that magical thinking—a coping mechanism. My last marriage dissolved within a year of the last blue moon on New Year's, the point at which I last became a vegetarian. Was I, as was Tesla, experiencing some sort of post-traumatic stress? Was I, by my heritage, predisposed to expect the worst? Would I become, as I had before in my previous marriages, what I had been as a child? Beaten down by the whips and opinions of others? Fat, sluggish, a non-entity? A waste, as my ex-husband at times insisted, of skin?

And the bigger question, first asked by the great singer Joni Mitchell, why do we dream in metaphor?

A relationship is a wilderness, whether it be with a dog, your own self, or another human. Walk through any wilderness while you are wearing blinders, and you are at least going to stub your toe, maybe break a leg or an arm, fracture a vertebra. In relationships, call them blinders of love and commitment. And so I found myself for the next few days stuck in a bloomless fog, feeling rejected and slighted over something unkindly said, a point Phil had tried to make about my writing habits being poorly executed. It had to do with what to me was work, but what to him was play because it didn't involve a salary. He didn't mean it the way he said it, but I believe strongly in the truth behind the Freudian slip. There's truth in every jest, an elder friend once told me. With the time the daily writing of this account was taking—writing that felt important to me because I was trying to understand where I was in my evolution in that moment, trying to understand the waxing and waning confusion I felt over how tired I was of juggling life alone—of doing it all—stacked against our impending marriage and a return to domestic life after having been so long single and independent, if often bored. And wondering, would I—could I—continue to *be* if I were once again a wife? A point I made clear to him over and over again: I'm a woman, and I will marry you, I want to be married with you, but I am not cut out to be a wife.

It was his call for attention, of course. Time spent on wedding preparations, Tesla, my job, and the writing—never mind the renovations, which had come to an apoplectic standstill after the great strides we'd made steaming off wallpaper in February—translated to Phil not getting the attention he needed at that moment in time, and, in truth, all because of complications the insertion of a dog had brought to our lives, at a time when his duties at work had burgeoned (translation: the American Recovery and Restoration Act of 2009, which was hell on federal contracting officers in 2010 when all that new money translated to new government contracts, and, according to Phil, would have little impact on actual economic recovery thanks to the amount of time it takes to get federal solicitations posted and contracts on the street and the dribbling way the work gets done and the slower dribble of getting people paid; but you never see one iota about that on our 24-7 newscasts).

I found myself wishing for the before. For all the entertainment a pet provides, it is, after all, very similar to adopting a child or having a baby, both of which require work and adjustment in catastrophic proportions. Adjustment which must be embraced, else all fail. To say I was tired is an understatement. To say I was dismayed over Phil's passive-aggressive jabs at me and not being better supported by my partner is another. Dinner that night ended up being vegetarian pizza at a restaurant neither of us liked. That I was beginning to feel very average when before I had felt magical, is an understatement, as well.

WANING CRESCENT MOON

WHEN ALL ELSE FAILS, COOK.

It was near the end of the semester, and I was preparing to travel again, this time for a week-long trip to Alaska for my very part-time job as a federal consultant in early childhood education. Not wanting to leave on bad terms, I came home on a late-April Thursday night, roughly one month before our wedding date, finally determined to mend whatever fences needed to be mended with Phil, to engage in the most healing endeavor I know and one I have come to realize is necessary for my spiritual and emotional well-being. I should not have been surprised by the greeting I received: Phil at the door with a ready hug, smiles, and a kiss, and Tesla on his hind legs trying to get his front paws around both of us after having spent a successful day in the crate. I have never felt as much love coming from an entity as was coming from that animal. Whatever was wrong, Tesla was trying to fix it. All the advice coming from all the corners about crating dogs was accurate. Was it possible Tesla was going to thrive from the security of the crate as much as he thrived from the exertion and exploration of our now daily treks? (I was reminded of the commitment to daily walking I'd made on New Year's. By acquiring Tesla, I had made that happen in spite of myself.)

And so the decision was made to advance to our local talking-it-all-out spot for some refreshment, with Tesla in tow. That perfect gentleman we'd glimpsed in the beginning had returned. He didn't mind sitting in Phil's little pickup, so long as he got to go, and I armed myself with little paw-shaped doggie treats to reinforce his good behavior every twenty minutes or so. I couldn't help myself in this regard, perhaps because it had brought about such success in his disciplining. Where before he used to run leaping to the sofa to watch Phil drive away in the mornings, now we walked Phil to the door. Tesla first was required to stay, then sit. After Phil left, Tesla got little doggie paw treats for complying. After several days of this, he was going straight to the pantry door where the treats lived and sat very prettily waiting for his reward, foregoing the sofa routine altogether. Very Pavlovian. And a relief.

However much stock a person puts into horoscopes doesn't matter to me. I believe all roads lead to home, but I am fond of Rob Brezny and his "Freewill Astrology," which is syndicated in alternative newspapers across the country and is available online. My Libra horoscope for that week advised me to begin thinking about my relationship with my significant other in terms of three—not insofar as dragging another human into our midst, but concerning the way I think of my relationship. That is, that the relationship itself is a third being on its own. We had talked about this, Phil and I, and we were both adult enough to realize that we must nurture the spirit of our joined selves much as we must nurture our bodies and, now, Tesla. Which is exactly what we did over a pair of pints that night, arriving, finally, at the source of Phil's consternation. I had to admit that my writing infiltrated our lives because I was doing it at our little breakfast table in the kitchen. This most recent jarring of his sensitivities had come about the previous Sunday morning as he was trying to serve me one of his spectacular breakfasts, to which I'd said, "Just let me finish this sentence." I didn't blame him. It probably would have unglued me, too, and we were still raw from the conflagration that, weeks prior, had landed us at the animal shelter eyeballing the part Plott's Hound/part Boxer we now loved and knew as Tesla.

Once again I listened to him explain how the American Recovery and Restoration Act of 2009 (ARRA) had his work life cranked to the same warp drive it reaches at the end of the fiscal year. Charged with spending government money wisely, he was one of the few gatekeepers for purchases or work requested by national parks within the western region of the U.S. (including Alaska and Hawaii).

Within certain dollar limits, project requests were apt to wind up on Phil's desk and had to be reviewed, approved, published, and the incoming proposals assessed for accuracy and ability before being chosen and the work overseen and paid for. He was trying to sort out the screwed-up writing messes people were submitting in the form of work and project requests. Phil hates bad writing. Raves about it. Preaches to the air about it. He doesn't want to put his name to a poorly written document, so he personally revises each work statement (multi-page documents required by law to be publicly posted so that the work may be fairly bid and so taxpayers may be guaranteed the "best value" for their spent dollars) before he posts it to the federal contracting website. Because ARRA funds were bonus dollars, people who normally didn't write project requests were worming their way out of the sheetrock, and Phil was faced with a mountain of poor writing at the same time as his superiors were saying, "Don't worry about it. It's good enough." And all the while I sat blithely tapping at the keyboard, writing stuff nobody ever may read. "It's wrong, and it's immature, but it's definitely making me feel disconnected from you," he said.

And I, of course, had a perfectly large and beautiful office space upstairs with decades of wallpaper slowly but definitely over the weeks now finally steamed off and the holes patched, waiting for new plaster and paint, the carpet ripped up, a new skylight and a new four by six window, shelves and shelves and shelves for all my books, a library table, a gorgeous computer armoire I bought and finished myself in such a way that it is always mistaken for an antique. So why was I holding court at the breakfast table?

It took me the entire next day to finally articulate yet another set of fears. I was as afraid of that lovely writing space as I used to be of a blank page. It was a marriage of its own kind. I was back to Tesla, again, so fearing the very thing he likely craved: food, warmth, and a safe place to be. That room upstairs was a manifestation of my oldest dream. Since my days of filling lock-and-key dime-store diaries, I had imagined an upstairs space with a skylight in which to do my writing. It had lodged in my memory the first time I read *Little Women*. I wanted to be Jo, to have that life of writing and the space in which to do it with an opening in the ceiling so I could look out at the stars at night, the blue and clouds and rain during the day. Now that it was mine, I didn't know what to do with it. A page of a catalog had come to life, but all I knew how to do was look at it. Stare at it. Wishing. Did I fear who I would be in that space? Fear the quality—or lack—of what would come when I conjoined with it? Or was it just that I was so accustomed to living without what I most desired? Like a dog who gets used to being balled up in a crate? Like a poor little country girl who spends her life staring at what can never be hers on the pages of the Sears catalog?

But. Always in life, I had been able to face what I feared, and surely this was no different. I would go forward in the direction I was headed. I would marry Phil. I would parent both him and Tesla when required, and they in turn would parent me. Phil was forcing me up those stairs, and I would go, lift the trowel, imagine myself Michelangelo, and sculpt new plaster over old, wetting the walls with a spray bottle as I went, letting the plaster free-form itself in the rough, old, mud tradition. I would make the process new and my own by layering bright colors of latex paint over it—blueberry, raspberry, chocolate, and putty-gray for the floors. I would wash the shelves and wood trim and give them a fresh coat of white. I would line up my armoire, haul upstairs the laptop and the printer, and go to work. I swore it to myself. I had many times talked to Phil long and hard about compartmentalizing his work so that he stopped bringing it home to dump onto our peace, so that we could while away our hours together in a relaxed state, renewing ourselves from the day rather than allowing it to leave its tread on us. I saw that he was asking me to do the same. I had trained him, and he had learned. He was asking me to leave work at work, where it belonged.

The meal that resulted from all this soul-searching and reconfiguring left us both twitching and moaning like happy dogs and, as Phil said, "Ain't bad for leftovers." The flavors intense and complicated, and for two people who can distinguish individual flavors, a field day. In that aspect it was among the most enjoyable meals we had yet created. Phil and I both love complicated flavor combinations, and in this case, we loved it so much we both went back for seconds and declared ourselves healed of all ills at the end of the meal.

Spicy Goulash

2 tablespoons extra virgin olive oil
2 tablespoons sunflower oil
1/2 red bell pepper, chopped
6 cloves garlic, minced
1 cup chopped celery
1 teaspoon dried basil
2 bay leaves
1 cup leftover Tesla's Rice
3 cups leftover Sweet Lentil Polou
Filtered water
1/4 teaspoon Tony Chachere's Original Creole Seasoning
Pinch dried red chilis
Sea salt to taste
Fresh ground black pepper to taste
1 cup Tillamook Vintage White Extra Sharp Cheddar Cheese
1 cup chopped bok choy
1/2 cup chopped leek

Combine oils in a large frying pan and sauté bell pepper, garlic, and celery over medium heat until partially soft. Add basil and bay leaves. Add leftover rice and polou and enough water to make a liquid mush. Bring to boil and cover. Simmer for 20-30 minutes or until all liquid is absorbed. Add seasonings to taste. Allow to rest, covered and with heat off, for 10 minutes. Add cheese and stir. Add leek and bok choy just before serving. Makes 4 large helpings.

* * *

Plaster's most engaging characteristic is that it is unforgiving. It forces a person to work methodically but quickly. Mistakes cannot be corrected since it cannot be sanded. From the time of mixing until it begins to set up is twenty minutes. All tools and mixing containers must be clean and free of previous plaster residue, else the hardening starts even sooner. If it is too set before it is troweled to the wall, it will drop off when it hardens. It helps to dampen the wall with a spray bottle before the slathering, or so I've found. Nobody told me I could sculpt texture directly onto a lathe and plaster wall, but I did know that a Venetian plaster finish involves mixing paint with plaster of paris, and that it can be done right on top of scored wallpaper, which I did two years ago on the wall behind the bookshelves in our upstairs guestroom. To me, it is a beautiful finish, and one that can still be repainted if desired. But the price of blending paint into plaster is more than either of us was interested in bearing. (A five by eight foot section cost roughly sixty dollars). And I didn't bother to investigate far enough to discover that sheetrock mud is actually the more inexpensive and practical substance to use. So it made sense to me to mix the plaster with water, sculpt the texture the way I wanted it, seal it, and then paint. Plaster mixed with water over paint is also much more pliable (read "playable") and looks a bit more rustic.

As much as I am drawn to primitive decor, I am also drawn to the finer things in life, so long as I can acquire them at a bargain price. Phil and I had two lovely Egyptian rugs on the wood floors downstairs. Tesla had chosen those as his spot to vomit daffodil and grass shoots. We bought the rugs at an auction when our local high-priced furniture store went out of business at a fraction of their five-hundred-dollar-apiece original price. I would never pay five hundred dollars for a rug. But I loved being able to describe them as "Egyptian." It appealed to my sense of the exotic.

To good food and its preparation I have to add hard work that enables a person to buy cool things as a mender of a disquieted mind. The end of a day where the human hand has met tools of labor and production is filled with tired grace. As I worked at the plastering, I was reminded of my brother Jacob and my father, both of whom had toiled long and hard in their lives, both of whom were gifted with the tools of carpentry. I don't know that I am so gifted, but I did love to imagine the long line of my genetics when I engaged my body in the physical way that plastering required. Many such a task I have tackled in my life, untrained, simply by saying to myself, if these generations of my family have done it, I must be able to, too. My heritage is one of problem solving by necessity. When every bite, every bit of shelter, every bit of luxury must proceed from your own body's ability to engage with what comes from the earth, you become inventive or you starve, or freeze, or learn to scavenge. I am thankful for days that remind me what it is to be alive in my body and less so in the mind. ("Are you perhaps too analytical?" asked my brother.) This balance is crucial for all of us, and we forget it in the chaos of our modern pace. My computer's screensaver at the time featured the words of Buddha: Chop wood; carry water. These are our only true duties.

We were talking about such things and the events of our day over a dinner of Phil's leftover Garden Lentil Soup, bolstered with shredded white cheddar, and even more Tony Chachere's. Phil's quote of the evening on our culture of the disenfranchised, promulgated, as he sees it, by the availability of junk food in America: "Why is there no place to which I can walk up and lay a nickel and buy a carrot?"

*   *   *

In trying to come up with an appropriate way to celebrate nearly four months of vegetarian living, Phil and I landed on hiking the trail at Nisqually John's Landing and preparing a complicated dish we'd been dreaming about but had been postponing for the sheer amount of time it took. Nisqually John's Landing is fourteen miles up the Snake River from Clarkston on the Lower Granite Reservoir, features a boat dock, and is the place where Phil, in 2007, was stricken with a hernia attack. Between his hernia operation and my knee surgery the next year, we hadn't been back since. The trail branches off the river road and winds up a lovely little basalt canyon that drops to a year-round creek flanked by burls of blackberry brambles, perhaps the closest place for us to pick blackberries not contaminated by vehicle exhaust.

Within a few minutes of having launched ourselves on the trail, we both spoke at once. The path was eerie in a way neither of us liked, filled us both with a sense of apprehension, much as making a decision to become vegetarian, take on a marriage, or a dog: who knows what cosmic comedy awaits? Judging from the stillness, which translated to the absence of bird or squirrel sounds, and the way Tesla launched maniacally against his leash trying to follow animal traces, we suspected we were in cougar territory. The air just had that feel about it. Phil and I had hiked through cougar country before, and we didn't think much of it. Having Tesla along was a bit of a reassurance, but only a bit. I did not relish watching the blood event of him trying to take down a cougar.

Although there was not one footprint and only one bit of curious scat, we both agreed we were likely being watched and were unsettled enough to consider cutting our outing short, until we heard the noise of other people at our tail, which went far toward calming our nerves. Nisqually John's had been featured in the newspaper the week before, so we had expected a stream of company and were surprised that it had taken so long to run across anyone. They passed us, and we felt secure enough to finish the hike. A cougar might pounce on a single human or a pair, but it was doubtful he or she would try to take on six. Besides, we could feed the cougar the scrawny college kids while we made our escape.

Similarly, I have no idea about how to comment on the return scene in the parking lot: a very large woman lying with her knees toward us in a gynecological position on an even larger, flat-topped boulder. We were both silent for the first half mile down the road until Phil and I simultaneously eyed each other sideways and started laughing hard enough that Tesla tried to nose his way between our seats and into the party. Some things are better left unsaid. What the hike proved to us was how much we'd changed since that maiden trip in 2007. And maybe that is what that bulbous parking lot maiden was meant to be: a symbol of what a lack of care can do to a person. Phil weighed a good twenty pounds less than he did at the time of his hernia attack. Since I don't weigh myself, I could only speak to the size of my clothing, which was down one size and working on the next. Our knees were more fragile, mine in particular, and neither of us could endure the down hills like we once did. We agreed that one of those devices that is part walking stick, part folding seat might come in handy for rest periods and decided we must invest in a set of trekking poles for each of us and that even knee braces might not be a bad idea. Such was the price we were paying for having survived into our fifties without having taken extraordinary care of ourselves.

Had we known, obviously, we might have conducted ourselves just a little bit differently.

The dish we wanted to try that evening was my own version of Lentil Nut Loaf from *Laurel's Kitchen*. We had left the lentils soaking for the two hours we were gone. It sounds a little strange, but the loaf is very dark and rich and cries out for gravy and mashed potatoes. We decided to stand in favor of no gravy and no starchy spuds, so we peeled lowly but tasty beets and boiled them for a side dish instead, alongside Phil's fabulous Hot and Spicy Stir-Fried Green Beans, so we could top the meal with a treat. He, for some reason, decided to buy a package of Newman-O's Hint O' Mint Cream Filled Chocolate Sandwich Cookies, so for dessert—chocolate teeth. We are great fans of Newman-O's Hint O'Mint Cream Filled Chocolate Sandwich Cookies, but even greater fans of Costco's Kirkland Brand frozen organic veggies, especially the green beans. We buy them in a five-pound bag, and if thrown frozen into first boiling water, then sieved immediately into hot oil, they cook as close to fresh as any either of us has ever tried. We make these last, after everything else is finished, so they can go straight from pan to table.

Neat Loaf

2 tablespoons sunflower oil
1 white onion, minced
1 tablespoon butter
2 cups French green lentils, cooked until very soft
1/2 cup hulled hemp seed
1/2 cup organic pretzels, finely ground
3/4 cup walnuts, toasted very dark
1/2 teaspoon ground thyme
3 tablespoons oat flour
1/2 cup vegetable broth
1/4 cup heavy cream or half-and-half
2 teaspoons organic white vinegar
2 teaspoons tamari sauce
Ketchup
2 eggs, slightly beaten
Toasted sunflower seeds, crushed

Preheat oven to 325 degrees. Sauté onion in oil until transparent and partially browned. Stir in butter until melted. Add all ingredients except eggs and sunflower seeds and mix well, then stir in eggs. Once the mixture is somewhat cool, pour into a buttered loaf pan. Bake, covered with foil, for 30 minutes or until set. Remove foil and sprinkle with sunflower seeds. Continue baking until browned around the edges and separated from the pan. Serve with mashed potatoes and gravy for a truly decadent main course.

Phil's Hot and Spicy Stir-Fried Green Beans

1/4 cup water
1 pound frozen Kirkland Organic Green Beans
2 tablespoons sunflower oil
Garlic granules
Salt
Fresh ground black pepper
Tony Chachere's Original Creole Seasoning

Heat water in wok or round-bottomed skillet over medium heat until very hot. Add beans and cook until water evaporates. Meanwhile, heat oil in a separate skillet. Sieve beans and drop into heated oil, stirring until evenly coated. Cook on medium-high heat, stirring occasionally, for 10 minutes or until edges of beans start to brown and crisp. Add liberal amounts of seasoning or to taste. Serve immediately.

*   *   *

We had a little undeclared competition in our house. It had to do with who was going to get to turn the calendar page when the new month rolled around. Neither of us had ever spoken a word about this or even breathed heavily while thinking about it in the presence of the other, but I could feel it, each time I remembered to do it before Phil did. It was this little look he got when he noticed I'd been there first. The slightest, tiniest, wince-like movement around the eye. I doubt anyone else could even see it. Perhaps this is why we had three calendars in our house, and most years four and five, if we remember to place one in the guest room upstairs. Earlier in the year, Phil was so intent on getting to the bathroom calendar first that he turned it after I'd already turned it, so it was a month ahead when I came in later. I didn't say a word, just chuckled to myself and fixed it. I loved being in the house with a man who cared about calendar pages. It told me he cared about time and the passage of time. Which meant he must understand and accept time's effect on him and me.

The March calendar page in the bathroom in 2010 had a photo of colored pencils arranged point-to-point, as if spokes on a wheel meeting at the hub or petals on a flower, and the large caption, "Balance." The caption for April was "Believe," for May, "Success." The night before we had made reservations for our honeymoon at a handful of excellent and mostly vintage hotels across Oregon. We planned to be in Baker City at the Geiser Grand Hotel Sunday night, the day after the wedding, then spend time in the Burns/Hines area, where I'd heard there was a burgeoning art scene, then Bend in the center of the state, and Yachats, on the coast, before arriving at our beachfront cottage on the northern coast at Oceanside to roost in front of the Pacific for three days. On night nine, we'd land in Walla Walla, Washington, at the Marcus Whitman Hotel, before coming home to spend a day regrouping then heading out to camp on the Lochsa River for the final few days.

Preparing for bed that night, I couldn't help but flip through those bathroom calendar pages thinking: this is good material for my share of the wedding vows and the plan and formula for the rest of our days: Balance + Believe = Success. Funny how sometimes drama leads us to awareness. If it weren't for the struggle of the previous weeks involving Tesla's misbehaving (he continued to destroy whatever he was left alone with, and he shat in my unfinished office!) arguments with Phil (he still couldn't understand why I wanted a prayer at our wedding, and considering his last wedding was Catholic, it seemed odd that he should object so vehemently to something so small, which, of course, made me suspicious that his struggle was about something else—cold feet perhaps?), grinding my way through end-of-semester grades, preparing now suddenly for an Alaska trip to do some consulting work, and the struggles with blood sugar, I wondered if I would have noticed those words on the calendar in the same way and what kind of impact they would have had. Everything happens for a reason, I'd heard myself saying to my brother Jacob over the phone. I had been reminding him how the little deaths that result from life's relatively minor traumas toughen our hides and prepare us to be able to perceive the bigger lessons when they come, as well as help to prepare us for that ultimate tragedy—the end of our physical existence.

*   *   *

Three times I have stood in front of a son and his wife listening to their proud but vaguely nervous testimony: We are pregnant! This time it was Jacob, my youngest, and his lovely wife Kelsey. ("Why don't you stop by today, Mom?" always tilts the cup of suspicion skyward just a bit.) They were expecting an October arrival, which meant, come fall, I would have grandchild birthdays to consider in January, May, and October. Add son birthdays in August and November and daughter-in-law birthdays in July and December and wedding anniversaries in June and February, and we had almost the entire calendar covered by next-generation celebrations. I needed a monthly gift and card budget—but I didn't mind.

I stood there listening to their proclamation feeling a distinct sense of disconnect. On the drive to their house I was consumed with thinking about how hard we'd been struggling with what to do about Tesla's diet. He was still eating grass, significant daily doses of it, which I'd learned is the way a dog settles his stomach. Translation: it settles his stomach because it is the doggie version of Syrup of Ipecac, that raunchy stuff we give people who've ingested something they shouldn't and therefore need to vomit. A dog's stomach then ejects the contents, which for Tesla, usually occurred as we were settling in for the evening, and the spot he kept choosing, as I've said, was the Egyptian rugs. That morning, however, he selected instead the cheap, dowdy runner in front of the kitchen pantry, a thing we'd both been aching to throw away as soon as we found an appealing replacement.

"I'm at the end of my ability to tolerate this," I had told Phil on the phone that morning, "I threw the stupid thing out. The rug, not the dog. But I'm putting you on notice. I've had enough. This dog has taken over my life. I can't get any work done."

"Well," he said, "we wanted to replace it anyway."

We'd heard just days before from friends about something called, in contradiction to itself, the BARF diet (for Biologically Appropriate Raw Food). The BARF diet is a simple return to the way dogs were fed up until the 1930s, when commercial dog food began to be produced—because it was the depression, and nobody was willing to spare people food, and it was a way of creating jobs—at which point the industry began its seduction of veterinary schools and their graduates, very similar to the pharmaceutical industry's seduction and brainwashing of today's medical schools and their graduates. Of course, with the widespread availability of glossy, commercial advertising, now the entire U.S. population is so seduced.

The BARF diet is easy and cheap and only requires engaging the local butcher shop or grocer's meat department to save for you their chicken necks and backs from naturally processed fowl. The purchase of a few naturally processed chicken wings might be required as a supplement (the kind raised with no hormones and no antibiotics). The dog gets a whole, raw egg three to five days a week. Ditto a little mackerel or a few sardines. Some advocates suggest adding a few raw vegetables. Big beef and pork bones with dabs of meat on them keep teeth serviced (dogs on the BARF diet never have to have their teeth cleaned) and jaw and chest muscles strong. What everyone seems to agree upon is this: no cooked anything; no grains of any kind; no kibble. Only a replication, or as close to as possible, of what canine ancestors would have once eaten in the wild. Phil questioned dogs in the wild finding eggs to eat. Some bird's nest on the ground, I told him. Mama for breakfast and eggs for dessert. "What dog doesn't love a henhouse?" I asked.

But for both of us, the jury was still out. We had to do more research. And we had already found testimony by the thousands, including the great zoo controversy. Apparently it is only in the United States that commercially prepared food is widely used in zoos.

By way of experiment, we did start Tesla with an eighteen-hour fast, and put a whole egg in his bowl on top of his kibble, which he first played with, then ate, with something akin to glee. Not much later, he was eating his morning dose of grass. Phil's comment on the BARF diet and on our noticing the very high grain content in most commercial dog food was this— "I've never seen a dog in a cornfield, except to chase a pheasant."

* * *

With so much of our time and energy being consumed by other things, we had yet to experiment with a wedding dessert line-up, in part, also, because neither of us cared overly much for dessert. Once in a while, however, we did get cravings for chocolate. From time to time we bought high-end organic chocolate and helped ourselves to one tiny square or two a night. The four ounce bar of chocolate-covered marzipan (with a tip of the hat to our dear friends, Lance and Andi—Lance introduced backwoods me to chocolate-covered marzipan during a graduate-level creative writing course in 1997; I believe at the time he explained to the class that there were really only two food groups: pizza and chocolate-covered marzipan) I bought Phil for Valentine's Day lasted a couple of weeks. And obviously I would never endorse a non-organic product without a supremely good reason, but earlier in April, beset with a hankering for chocolate-chip-oatmeal cookies that absolved itself before I reached the front door on my return home, I picked up a package of Albertsons' Essensia brand chocolate chips because of its short list of ingredients. It sat in the pantry for a while, until we started pilfering from it. To be succinct, they were the best chocolate chips I'd ever tasted coming out of a grocery store, and they lasted on the tongue just long enough to satisfy even intense chocolate desire, before melting into perfect, soul-gracing, chocolate oblivion. Likewise, I very rarely bought dried fruit, because organic dried fruit was expensive, and non-organic brands kept their pretty up by using sulfite preservatives, which gave me headaches.

But on that same shopping trip I discovered Mariani dried fruits out of Vacaville, California. They are not an organic food company, but they use no preservatives save a bit of sugar and are an old establishment founded on certain standards of quality the family still maintains over a hundred years later. They are, in fact, the largest dried fruit company in the world, and for good reason: they sell a very high-quality, minimally processed product. I bought their cherries, pineapple, and tropical fruit and fully admit they were tasty and satisfied a sweet tooth, which is why I never got around to making the oatmeal cookies: I sampled the pineapple on the way home. Dried fruit is great nutritious stash food and especially convenient to have on hand for hiking and travelling, although obviously calorie-dense, so use it judiciously. The dessert gorp we made that one night (to top off Phil's very excellent Asian-meets-Creole dish, Spring Fever) from that collection of otherwise unused ingredients, might as well have been heroin. Elegant Dessert Gorp should be declared a drug and to consume it, pure hedonism. There should be an award for anyone who can stop at only one handful. Be careful with the Spring Fever; it will melt your earwax. And be warned: the meal renders a person fit for nothing but the couch and the remote control.

Spring Fever

2 cups uncooked brown basmati rice
1 tablespoon olive oil
1 medium zucchini
1 pound asparagus
2 tablespoons sunflower oil
1/3 cup yellow onion, chopped
1 1-inch piece ginger root, peeled and minced
1 red bell pepper, cut into 1-inch pieces
1 cup red cabbage, chopped
1 teaspoon crushed red pepper
1/2 teaspoon fresh ground black pepper
1 teaspoon garlic granules
1 tablespoon Trader Ming's Soyaki (from Trader Joe's)
1 teaspoon Tony Chachere's Original Creole Seasoning
Cashews, roasted

Bring 4 cups water and olive oil to a boil in a medium saucepan. Add rice, then lower heat and cover. Simmer for 45 minutes or until done. (Rice may be cooked ahead and then refrigerated until needed.) Cut zucchini in half lengthwise and then into half-inch slices and set aside. Cut asparagus into 1-inch slices then steam until still crunchy but not raw and set aside. Heat sunflower oil in a large wok or round-bottomed skillet over medium high heat until extremely hot. Add onion, ginger, and red bell pepper and cook, stirring constantly, until translucent. Add asparagus, zucchini, and cabbage, stirring constantly, until cabbage and asparagus become bright in color. Stir in crushed red pepper, black pepper, and garlic. Add rice and stir. Add Soyaki, then season to taste with creole seasoning. Top each serving with a generous handful of roasted cashews. Makes six generous portions.

Elegant Dessert Gorp

1 cup Mariani Dried Cherries
1/2 cup Essensia Real Semi-Sweet Chocolate Chips
1 cup raw almonds

Toast raw almonds at 325 degrees for 2 hours or until the skins just start to darken. Allow to cool, then chop very coarsely. Combine all ingredients thoroughly. Add extra chocolate chips if desired. Makes 10 quarter-cup servings.

* * *

I breakfasted rather sinfully on the last of the Elegant Dessert Gorp one morning while checking email. Even though I was happy to hear from Jill Nugent, who continued to follow the situation in Haiti, once again I found my largess juxtaposed against the inelegance of life in Haiti:

"Dear friends of Haiti—as I prepare for my annual trip to the island of La Gonave in Haiti, some things feel the same, and some things feel very different. I know that there will be a warm and joyous reception from my Haitian friends and colleagues and that while there, I'll help move grassroots projects forward however I can; however, the whole context will be different in the aftermath of the earthquake. Another thing that will really be different is that three people from Moscow, Idaho, will be coming with me to experience Haiti for themselves, and the four of us are backed by tremendous support from friends and strangers who have reached out to Haitians at this time. The level of support is astonishing and wonderful. So many thank yous are in order: for financial and emotional support, and for the efforts of so many people who made the Breakfast for Haiti Fundraiser a success last month. That event raised about $7,000. Since the earthquake, we've received $15,000 in donations to the effort to "help Haitians improve their lives on their own terms." This work felt huge before the January 12th disaster and continues all the same. I am honored to be the go-between. Although La Gonave didn't experience the widespread death and devastation of the cities, it has absorbed thousands of injured, displaced and traumatized people. We are supporting communities that are generally neglected by the large aid machine, communities that (sadly) have a lot of experience with making do after political and natural catastrophes. They will try to parley every nickel into getting work done in ways that address long-term problems and build sustainability. The big issues right now are adequate food, planting season (now), repairing/rebuilding homes, post-traumatic stress, school for the many new children, overcrowded houses. The groups I'm connected to are working out stopgap measures for the most dire situations while making assessments and working out long-term strategies. I'll know more details after the trip."

*   *   *

By that first week in May, mere days before my last minute trip to Alaska, we started to see amazing changes in Tesla, which we attributed to the introduction of raw food into his diet. He was no longer just sleeping at night; he vanished into sleep. What follows is a very small sampling of the stunning number of testimonies from e-communities (such as dogmagazine.net) devoted to the growing population of dog and cat owners who have switched their pets to the BARF diet. *Give Your Dog a Bone* by Australian veterinarian Ian Billinghurst is the book that sparked the movement in the early '90s. Anyone who decides to research this diet for his or her own pets should strictly avoid the sites that are trying to sell "raw" meat products for dogs. Capitalism ever blooms.

- "My poor pooch had horrible hot spots from constant chewing of her paws. I tried everything from hypo-allergenics to hot sauce but no luck. A friend of mine told me about the BARF Diet, and we gave it a shot. I was amazed to see Claire not only stop chewing but regain her lost youth! It really is amazing stuff and well worth the money!"

- "My Tibetan Terrier, Chewy, used to be a VERY picky eater. I tried so many different brands of kibble and canned food but he still would not eat. He also suffered from diarrhea and other digestive issues from the constant changes in his diet. A friend of mine suggested that I try BARF. Chewy absolutely loves this food! He's gained some much-needed weight and no longer has digestive issues. Plus, his breath is much better and his teeth are cleaner after being on the BARF diet for about a year."

- "After switching my French bulldog, Peanut, to a raw food diet two years ago, I've noticed serious improvements in her health. . . . I've learned that a diet consisting of just raw meat, vegetables, and vitamin supplements is the best meal you can feed your pet. Peanut had endless problems prior to the raw food diet; yeast infections, hot spots, pancreatitis, but since switching her to raw foods she's been in much better health."

- "I put my cat on a raw food diet a little over two years ago. He has diabetes and had been very sick, and I thought I was going to lose him. Since the prescription cat food didn't seem to be helping him, I took matters into my own hands. I figured, if nothing else, he would enjoy his food for the last few weeks of his life. What a

turnaround! He got better and is now playful and healthy—
people can't believe he's sixteen years old! His diabetes is
under control, and I don't think he's ever been happier."

- "We work closely with a small, private shelter in Derbyshire.
  The people who run the shelter followed our suggestion
  and took on the BARF diet for one of the young dogs at
  the shelter whose behavior was so atrocious that people
  would sidle gingerly past her enclosure when they were
  viewing dogs. No one in their right mind would want
  Sasha in their home. Because she was housed in a kennel
  with a cement floor, she was deprived of her ability to
  forage and supplement her diet. Also, the stress factor
  associated with kenneling further depleted her of vital
  nutrients. She consequently became unmanageable in
  her desperation to supplement and survive. Her behavior
  changed dramatically with proper feeding and Sasha is
  now happily doing much better. After this experience,
  the shelter gradually adopted the BARF diet for all of the
  rescue dogs in the shelter. Their feeding and veterinary
  expenses have markedly reduced and the previously
  unwanted dogs are being picked very quickly. It is easy
  to re-home a placid, well-behaved dog."

- "Stroller, a fourteen-month-old Blue Roan Cocker Spaniel
  was scheduled for destruction when the owner contacted
  us. He had attacked his owner. In unraveling the story,
  we found that Stroller had jumped up on the table, snatched
  a tissue and run under the table guarding his trophy
  aggressively. What Stroller didn't know was that the
  owner's engagement ring was inside the tissue. She
  naturally went under the table to retrieve it and Stroller
  attacked her. She was heartbroken because she thought
  that Stroller had turned on her. One of the first things we
  noticed about him was the putrid smell from both ends.
  This is one of the signs of dietary stress that we look for.
  We started him on the BARF diet immediately. Over the
  next four weeks, the smell disappeared and so did his

aggressive possessiveness with items. He took naturally to the diet as do most dogs and that, with a combination of training, exercise and manipulation, produced an absolute treasure of a dog that anyone would be proud to own. He doesn't now need to 'hunt' to supplement his diet, as he was doing when he snatched the tissue. It would have been so easy to destroy him for his 'aggressive' behavior."

* * *

"Never place blame on the porcupine who was not born to see beyond the length of his quills."

—Old Native American saying

The day before my departure to Alaska started with Phil stir-frying fresh, local, organic vegetables for lunch later in the day and at the same time working on the *Moosewood Cookbook's* Eggplant Parmesan for dinner. (Not supper, as I grew up calling it in Indiana.) I had also spent time on the phone listening to Mom, who was reporting on Dad's efforts at building a bonfire. He'd been dragging stuff into a pile in the driveway's dirt turnaround off and on ever since I'd left, she said. *Good,* I thought but did not say. *Exercise.*

Our Saturday morning ritual involved a trip to pick up coffee, after which we sat and read the paper. Scones were in order on this particular Saturday, since the next day it was *bon voyage*. The Lewis-Clark Valley was in early bloom, the violet of ornamental plums abundant. The Snake and Clearwater Rivers were the color of foil again.

We wanted to enjoy our morning, but we couldn't really. We had to address the drama that was Tesla. We were running out of time. I was leaving for a week. I'd be back two weeks and then the wedding. Our backyard fence, which before I left for Mom and Dad's back in March had begun to look like a scary redneck's bad art, by the beginning of May looked like camouflage for a moonshiner: junk boards and discarded particle board shelves and bits of fencing nailed to what was once pretty white lattice framed in dove gray.

Now it was an atrocity, to which Tesla's response had been simply to jump the four-foot fence on the other side of our lot. He'd been making his way to a neighbor's house each morning where boxer cousins resided, so sadly, we decided to chain him to a runner. He now had thirty feet of tether attached to an overhead cable which ran from the house to a post the previous owners had set—likely for the same purpose. Of course, during the hours we were gone on Friday, Tesla had wreaked havoc within that thirty-foot radius—snapped tulip stems, ripped out rock, crushed established shrubs, mangled yard art, chewed on deck boards.

The BARF diet may have cured his grass eating and his skin lesions—those things we at first thought were alley-fight wounds—and he may have been sleeping better, but he was also much more energetic.

Phil finally declared that he'd had enough. All week long he had made daily calls into the animal shelter, waiting for a spot to open up so we could return the dog. It was at once a heartbreaking choice and a relief.

Equally as sad, however, was the fact that Phil, in looking for a place to put his anger, had decided to blame the entire situation on my lack of patience. And it was true. I had no patience for an animal tearing up the place, no matter how much I loved him. My brother Jacob, too, insisted the dog was acting on my vibes. "What is this blaming business," I asked them both. "How is it me and my lack of patience that's the problem? The dog is clearly in the wrong environment. Why does it have to be anyone's fault? Why can't it just be that we got a lemon?"

What I haven't explored much here is the voice. The voice of Tesla. A whining wail that sounded like a woman in pain. For hours on end. Any time and for the entire time we left him alone, according to Paul, our neighbor to the north. As a woman who spent decades looking for permission to have a voice, the last thing I wanted to do was to complain about and shut down someone/something else's. But shut it down we did. Before we even got a dog, Phil and I had had discussions about those awful surgeries that cancel out a dog's bark. We'd always agreed it was criminal. Now, we concluded, we'd begun to understand it.

And so later that afternoon, I pulled out my wallet yet again and bought a muzzle and a ten-foot tether, so far-reaching was the state of destruction upon having returned from work that Friday evening and so tangled was the dog. We were lucky he hadn't hanged himself. What a sorry state of affairs.

But at least those accoutrements kept Tesla quiet enough for me to do some yard work. Hands in the dirt, wielded pruning shears. Lop. Lop. How good it felt to be focused on ridding at least our immediate landscape of lunatic excess. Spring had made its display, living green coming back in doubles and triples. The root of one shrub we both despised took over half an hour to dig up—a big, sunshine-yellow thing stark enough to make dye. The sound of the maddox hitting it was the sound of metal on stone. Tesla stood guard, rewarding me for my effort by climbing all sixty pounds of himself onto my lap and laying his head on my chest in odd juxtaposition to what was now two months of crazed behavior.

Phil's response to the pain of the situation was to go for a haircut and a summery dye job of his own. *Just lighten the tips, please.* Then he came home and created the very crunchy East Meets West Burritos (why is chewing so satisfying?) and all was right with the world, for a few moments.

East Meets West Burritos

> 1 15-ounce can New Directions Pinto beans
> 1 15-ounce can New Directions Black beans
> 1 tablespoon garlic granules
> 1-2 jalapenos, finely diced
> 1/2 cup chopped onions
> 1-1/2 cups cooked white basmati rice
> Don Pancho's Gordita-style Burrito Tortillas
> 1 head endive, chopped
> 1-1/2 cups bok choy, shredded
> Toasted sunflower seeds
> Kirkland Mild Organic Salsa
> Tillamook Shredded Mexican Blend Cheese (cheddar,
>   Monterey Jack, Queso, and Asadero version)

In a large skillet over medium heat, mash, stir, and cook
beans, garlic, jalapenos, and onion. Layer beans and rice
in flat tortillas with small portions of remaining ingredients.
Fold over ends and roll into burritos. Serves six.

*   *   *

The final straw came when the police called Phil at work a week
later, the day I was due back from Alaska, saying that someone had
called in to complain yet again about the animal being chained and
crying like he was wounded. Apparently they'd had several complaints
during the week, but when the patrol officers drove by our house
after those calls, they didn't hear Tesla, so they didn't call us. On
Friday, we weren't so lucky. Their message to Phil: You are going to
have to do something about that animal.

According to the tearful story Phil relayed that evening, he had
immediately called the animal shelter and, finally, they had an opening.
He said he'd taken off from work, driven home to find Tesla so
snarled in the chain he wouldn't have survived the afternoon but still
with space enough for his pharynx to generate that screaming, ice-
pick-in-the-shower, falsetto wail. Phil explained how he'd felt the
deaths of all the dogs he had ever lost rushing out of him as he'd
bawled in front of a room full of clerks and animal caregivers at the
shelter. How he'd yelled at them, saying they should do a better job
of communicating a dog's temperament before letting people lay
down their hearts and cash for them.

I don't know how long Phil cried that day in front of those people,
I've never asked, but I'm pretty sure it closely equaled the amount of
tears that quite literally burst forth from me when I arrived home to
the news. It hurt in that way it hurts when someone you love is
suddenly dead.

We sobbed into the dusk, not giving a thought toward eating dinner.

* * *

Our grieving was thankfully interrupted the next day by another unplanned—but this time welcome—event: the late-Saturday-evening arrival of Sean, Susannah, Malory, Leah, and their English springer spaniel, Molly, who so adored Phil and was so attuned to him that she'd start dancing around the back of the family's SUV as soon as they approached the interstate bridge between Lewiston and Clarkston. They listened to our woeful tale, offered jokingly to let Phil take temporary ownership of Molly—in other words, to dog-sit for a while. Sean was dropping Susannah and the girls at Susannah's mother's house in Moscow for the week. He'd return for them all the following Friday.

It was an idea neither of us rejected.

What a joyous Sunday spent with them and what a comfort as we experienced being released from weeks and weeks of stress. Pajamas and coffee until noon, Malory at the coffee table with water color pencils and a new, over-sized princess coloring book. A girl who usually started her day wearing a ball gown over PJs, Malory loved everything "Princesses," and whined because Susannah hadn't brought a dress for her to wear that morning. Poor child, forced to wear jeans the entire day. Where her sister loved the freedom of flowing skirts, Leah, now ten weeks old, preferred the confinement of swaddling. Eventually I sent Sean and Susannah out to the store for walnuts, spinach, and mozzarella, the only lasagna ingredients I was missing, and which I'd planned for the night's meal. Phil was making a run to the plant nursery for dozens of white petunias we hoped would be bursting forth by the time our wedding date arrived. It was my first tour of duty alone with two grandchildren. Leah napped to Mozart while Malory and I dosed tomatoes with sautéed vegetables and spices. She decided it was easier to dump spice from the small bail-lidded jars rather than spoon it, so the mix was out of balance, but who cared? Would anyone notice the half-cup of dried parsley versus the usual quarter cup? Two teaspoons of basil versus one? "The Beautiful Way," she termed our backyard, and stopped during her spice-dumping chores to stare at it from her perch on our 1950s ladder stool. "I can see The Beautiful Way from here, G-ma," (pronounced

jee-ma; a label I chose for myself before she was born, and which stuck)
she said, "I can really see it."

Sean and his family left Sunday afternoon, and I was glad we
had their dog Molly to smooth the void left by Tesla, especially for
Phil. The relief for me very quickly overpowered the grief. But he
was suffering through old psychology the experience had dredged
up, spent the waning hours of the afternoon trying to dig out old
poison in the form of digging spots in the earth for all those white
petunias. The great fireball of emotion stilled when he came into the
house to share with me the hawk feather he'd found lying next to
Tesla's teddy bear in the far back of the yard near the chain-link dog
run over which Tesla so expertly vaulted early in his time with us.

Moments later, a flock of perhaps forty cedar waxwings swooped
down upon our back yard. In fifty-three years of living, I had never
seen a flock of cedar waxwings. I had never seen a single cedar waxwing.
They were masked, like exotic bandits, with two black, connected
triangles around their eyes. Their color otherwise was a hazy blend of
pale gray and taupe, tails dipped in flamboyant sun yellow, spots of
cardinal below where each wing intersected with the body. They
migrate along waterways in search of berries, and our location here
at the confluence of two great rivers was a likely place for them, but
they usually wintered down along the California coast, and we were
very far inland, plus it was too early for them to be so far north.
Whether they are normal visitors to the Lewis-Clark valley, I can't say,
but to us, their presence there, at that time, was magical and odd. The
spirit that was Tesla had become a lesson for our lives, and this flock
of exotic-looking birds somehow his gift to us. "He knew he was
going to leave," I heard myself say to Phil. "That's why he climbed
into my lap that night before I left for Alaska." We both felt as if we
had been caught and released by something. But what? And why?

* * *

Peace. This was what peace felt like. How had I, in seven short
weeks, forgotten? Because they weren't short, that is why. Stressful
periods are never short in terms of their effect on your heart, mind,
and body. All day the first day I heard the jingle of doggy ID tags. Of
course it was the wind chimes responding to the bit of breeze cast

upon us to augment the white-cloud-blue-sky day, but my mind went to doggy ID tags. Phil had taken the day off Monday, and we had decided to leave the house early to get away from the sound of such ghosts and the sense we both had that Tesla was pining for us. Translation: we were pining for him.

Along the Snake River for thirty or so miles, then the Grande Ronde. A pickup full of large driftwood scavenged along the way from which Phil planned to sculpt flower beds before the wedding. A productive, relaxing morning followed by a frustrating afternoon as he tried to make the odd-shaped pieces work in conjunction with the great roots of our backyard's sixty-foot sycamore. Throughout the day, we grieved off and on in our various ways. For Phil, tears at the sight of Tesla's pile of chewed and now weathering bovine leg bones. For me, grief as fatigue; my afternoon raking and pruning interrupted by long pauses and periods of sitting in a yard chair to stare into space from behind polarized shades. We reasoned with each other as the day passed, remarking on how much we did not understand that Tesla had become our relationship. We agreed that neither of us understood how big a wedge his care had been, how much we did not ever want such a wedge again. Then, the day's only highlight: telling the stories about my trip to Alaska and giving up Tesla to my father over the phone, and hearing him laugh.

What I wanted otherwise of that day was nothing. I wanted no dishes in the sink, no laundry piles, no yard work, no plastering and painting still to be done, no wedding pending. I wanted a good book and the sofa. Why was that such a tough donation to make to myself? The weather swooped down to favor me in the form of blasting wind gusts and pummeling drizzle, like little needles piercing the skin. Nothing to do but go inside.

When it became clear the book reading would turn into a nap, I made myself rise and attend to shopping and dinner duties instead, lest I wake feeling worse. Out in the world, the work of spending money. Bills, groceries, odd housewares from discount stores (a pizza stone for four dollars and ninety-five cents!). It all added up to a day spent. At four-fifteen, inexplicably overcome by guilt and without premeditation, I phoned the animal shelter with all the Tesla instructions I could think of, including how we had healed his sores with the BARF diet. Trying with all my heart to make up for the defeat, the shirking of duty, the failure I felt.

*   *   *

The advantage of being older is that emotional pain does not last as long as it did in youth. The years teach a person to endure and heal as quickly as possible. So it was that Phil and I at mid-week found our way, once again, to our favorite talking-it-out spot, the Riverport Brewery, to eat popcorn and let ourselves be soothed by our favorite local manifestations of creative hops chemistry: my River Rat Red to his Cedar Rock Pale Ale. We noted how great it felt to leave Molly behind knowing she'd do nothing to upset her environment, then spent several hours recapping "The Experience that was Tesla," as we'd labeled it, finally deciding once again that there was nothing else we could have done, that Tesla needed a wider berth than we could offer him. Emotion had also been stirred for me that Tuesday by two gorgeous Alaskan huskies another instructor was trying to house in the office next to mine. Where they usually were calm and easily remained in her office for several hours while she taught, that day they had been intent on clawing down that state-funded door. I assumed they were catching my torn-up vibe. Another instructor had stopped to share her shelter-dog tale, but in her story, the dog "adjusted" after almost a year, and now they were happy they'd kept him. "You should watch Marley and Me," she said, but I knew there was no way I was going to. I knew the storyline well enough to know they kept that dog and lived with his indelicate idiosyncrasies and chronic—if innocent—destructive habits.

I'm amazed at what folks endure until their dogs "get it," including vomiting and nerve-induced diarrhea—as Sean and Susannah did with Molly—and the absolute certainty that dogs are humans born to live in human houses and be treated as dignitaries. I simply must be missing that gene. I can endure a great amount, but not doggie effluvia. Truth told, Tesla lost me the first night I got up to use the bathroom and stepped in doggie vomit, which was the day before he shit his crate the first time.

There is a haunting line in the film Rob Roy, spoken by Jessica Lange's character after having been raped by her husband's unscrupulous political aggressor, played by Tim Roth: "That which cannot be helped, must be endured." That sentence stuck with me, and has gotten me through some difficult times, spells of years when I felt I had no supporters, when all were at odds with what I knew to be my own worth. Life—and the "mistakes" I've made—have taught me to endure. It's not a bad skill to have, and I doubt a person can make it to eighty without it. Tesla, I understood, was just another bump in the road, one that revealed to me another truth about myself, and that is that I have no tolerance for pets. I'd rather be at the swimming pool, in the weight room, plastering, painting, raking, and, above all else, working on my most current writing project. I'd rather be spending my money on clothing and trinkets for my grandchildren or buying a plane ticket home to tend to my parents and their difficulties, not paying vet bills or buying elaborate electric collars and robot fences to keep an animal contained and quiet. Let that animal be free. Let me be free. Some people need and are up to the challenge. My totem animal, as declared by several Nez Perce and Coeur d'Alene folks, is the wolf, emblem to native cultures of the storyteller. Perhaps that is the problem. I doubt a wolf would have much patience for a relative who did not know how and when to shut up, sit down, be still, and listen.

Phil and I used eating as a means of dealing with the change in our household dynamic. He woke up that Friday, the Friday before our wedding week, with a stabbing eye pain, a sign he had sinus congestion and impending infection and reason enough to stay home from work and drink mullein tea. Unfortunately, or fortunately, it was my day to work from home, which meant I had to transfer my office to the coffee shop for a while.

After a couple of hours of revision work on my novel manuscript, I returned home to find Phil showing signs of recovering. We didn't really have time to take a day off, but we did, and so an afternoon of movies and food commenced: *Blind Side* and *Old Dogs*, two heart-warming films we both enjoyed; organic pretzel sticks from Costco with Beaver State Chinese Mustard/Extra Hot; leftover lasagna; leftover cornbread; granola bars; hemp shake; jalapeno cheese toast; tortilla chips and salsa; candy-coated sunflower seeds; and, somewhere in there, I had my morning bowl of oatmeal.

It was not a pretty sight.

I've come to recognize that Phil occasionally nosedives into a "Scorpio declivity" as I now think of it; a.k.a., he vanishes into a psychic cave for a couple of days, eats everything he can get his hands on, watches a half dozen or so movies, and then comes out the other side — as if he were living in his own chick flick. I don't normally join him, but this time I did, after three o'clock or so, anyway. I did have a quantity of work to finish. But by three-thirty, I was making the run to the movie store, shoring myself with Goetze's Caramel Creams, a soft caramel chew surrounding a fondant center I used to crave as a kid and have not tasted since I left my Indiana childhood behind. For some reason, they have begun appearing on store shelves here in the Lewis-Clark Valley, and I have had to avoid them for fear the eleven-year-old in me is quash-proof. Suffice it to say, with that bit of kick-start, I had joined the day's food fest. Neither of us could now quote how many calories we'd consumed, but it was too many to make any kind of yard work comfortable. Funny that we should use food as our drug, considering how much of a role diet had played in our lives with Tesla. It pained me to know he was right back on that famous expensive dog food, the brand most commonly donated to the animal shelter and that had him covered in sores when he dropped into our lives.

* * *

Going to lunch with work colleagues as a way of closing out the semester and saluting my upcoming wedding meant having to explain the fact that I had become a vegetarian. Being good liberals, they were, of course, equal parts curious and supportive. It's not quite the same as admitting you've become Christian, or Buddhist, or decided to move to India, but the inclination to assume a defensive posture was for me the same. It had to do with the fact that some of these same work colleagues knew that just a few years ago I was touting the advantages of a high meat-based protein diet as a way to recover from systemic candidosis, which meant I also had to explain how I had finally been able to overcome this life-altering condition. By some accounts, systemic candidosis is a silent epidemic in a world where antibiotics are handed out like gumdrops, an action often ensuing solely from a phone conversation with a physician.

I can remember dozens of times when I would awake with a sniffle and my mother would call our family doctor for penicillin, the only doctor in the small rural village of Lanesville, Indiana, near where for seven years (beginning when I was two) we lived in a basement without a house. Residing in basements in that day and place was a not-uncommon way to have your cake and eat it, too. To escape the confines of city dwelling, folks sunk a cement box partially into the ground against the day when they would finally have enough cash on hand to start buying two-by-fours and framing a house. It wasn't a bad way to go, I suppose, but we never quite got around to the house part, and our basement, being halfway underground, or *bermed*, was dark and damp, and the coal oil heater we used to keep us warm made me wake up with black snot or gave me sneezing fits in the middle of the night. Mom equated this with a cold and cranked the handle on the telephone to call the doctor for penicillin, which a few days later would always arrive in the mail.

The problem with antibiotics, of course, is that they don't work on cold viruses; meantime, they kill off those good bacteria known as your protective micro-flora. Everyone is born with his or her own batch, and if it gets killed off, it is very shy about coming back. Now, of course, we know you must repopulate those dead micro-flora, or another army will take over: yeast, the enemy of humans. It proliferates in intestines digging its way out through microscopic holes until it eventually infiltrates the entire system. Dysbiosis, as it is known, was first recognized in Japan in nursing home patients who, after consuming sugar, not only appeared drunk but had alcohol in their bloodstreams without having taken a drop of it. I suffered for years with dysbiosis in the late 1980s through the 1990s before learning about it from an astute pharmacologist who had been handing me repeat six-week courses of one of the strongest antibiotics available at the time to treat chronic sinus infection. He was also the one who suggested I might be allergic to cow's milk, not just lactose intolerant, but allergic to, obviously, whatever the cow had been eating prior to being milked—which more than likely included some sort of artificial feed designed to spike milk production. Suspending milk consumption was easy, and it took many years, but eventually I was able to resume using small amounts of milk product (I must have cream in my coffee, as I believe I've stated, else the lack will surely kill me)—until, of course, I started developing those dad-blamed ear infections.

Getting rid of the yeast was not so easy, nor was repopulating my intestine. It took thirteen years or so, the first two of which were riddled with doses of a powerful oral antifungal called fluconazole, or Diflucan, which at that time was mostly used intravenously for treating AIDS patients. Fluconazole is commonplace today, as is knowledge of systemic candidosis. But at that time the subject was a dark hole and finding a physician who knew how to treat it was impossible unless you went to a large city. Fortunately, I had a physician friend who was willing to let me, as a nurse, do my own research, and based on which he was willing to treat me. I believe I was on nearly weekly doses of Diflucan for over a year. I don't know how many liver function tests I had to have because of it. We just couldn't get the yeast to stay down. Unfortunately, I also had to give up my vegetarian diet, since yeast must be starved by avoiding carbohydrates, on which they feed. Treatment included six months of nothing but meat and boiled vegetables. I grew thin as a rail, "model thin" one friend called me. I swallowed acres of probiotics. For more than a decade after, I avoided carbohydrates as much as possible. To consume them meant to blow up like a tractor tire. It was an awful battle, and I constantly was trying to ward off my own cravings and my own innate way of being. I ate meat and cans and cans and cans of tuna. I fell off the wagon. I got back on. And continued to swallow dozens and dozens of bottles of probiotics, which were doing me little good because few probiotics can survive the hydrochloric acid bath they are exposed to in the stomach. Luckily, in the meantime, a few manufacturers began producing enteric-coated probiotics, and I discovered fasting. I found the combination of an occasional fast and an occasional bottle of high-quality enteric-coated probiotics eventually pulled me the rest of the way out of that horrible cycle, which is why I was finally able once again, to return to a meatless diet.

Signs and Symptoms of Dysbiosis:

- Chronic digestive complaints including gas, bloating, cramping, thrush (overgrowth of candida in the mouth), and rectal itching

- Chronic fatigue
- Recurrent vaginal or urinary infections
- Food/environmental allergies
- Low immune function
- Severe PMS
- Loss of libido
- Depression/anxiety
- Respiratory problems
- Prostatitis
- Sensitivity to perfumes and chemical smells
- Spaciness

Possible Causes or Contributing Factors:

- Prolonged antibiotic use which kills the good bacteria, allowing yeast overgrowth
- Oral contraceptive use, estrogen-replacement therapy, and/or steroidal use (Yeast festers in estrogen)
- Anti-ulcer medications including Zantac and Tagamet (reduction in hydrochloric acid lowers natural defenses to infection by enteric pathogens)
- Immune suppression due to stress, environmental toxins, illness and infectious agents
- Poor dietary habits, including high sugar intake
- Chemical/environmental toxins
- Alcohol use (alcohol is very toxic and feeds the yeast)
- Food and environmental allergies
- Hypothyroidism
- Diabetes (candida thrives in the presence of sugar)

- Gallbladder problems (parasites especially will hinder the production of bile and hydrochloric acid as will enzymatic deficiencies)

- Hypoglycemia and/or hypoadrenia

- Impaired liver function (The liver is a key organ in fighting against candida, since it is essential in detoxifying the toxins released when killing off yeast. If the liver is not strong enough to filter the blood, the toxins will remain in the blood and cause symptoms to become worse.)

- Mercury amalgam dental fillings

*   *   *

It had been one of those days. The kind where a person insignificant to your life, or a virtual stranger, says just the right incorrect thing, and the next thing you know you have found yourself a quiet place to do a little crying. In this case, I was in downtown Lewiston, looking for shoes to go with the wedding dress I had found en route to Alaska. It was one of our neighborhood homeless schizophrenics who yelled from across the street that I should consider going on a diet. As if I'd never thought of it myself.

Crying is good for the body. It has the same effect as eating a bar of chocolate or running a mile or two. It causes a release of endorphins. Which is why, I believe, people become addicted to feeling bad. Some of my favorite quotes on crying—all from unknown authors:

- "Who does not weep with his whole heart neither knows how to laugh."

- "If you're going to make me cry, at least be there to wipe away the tears."

- "If someone hurts you, cry a river, build a bridge, and get over it."

- "If someone hurts your feelings, shame on both of you."

THIRD QUARTER MOON

"A man's home is wherever he prospers."

—Aristophanes

AH, THE FRENZY OF ACTIVITY AROUND COMPANY. We had decided early on that we would be selective about who conducted our wedding ceremony. We did not want to be married by some random church pastor. We wanted someone who cared about us. Those two things are not necessarily mutually exclusive, but in our case, we simply didn't know any ministers, and we didn't want a stranger overseeing our day. And so, after some heart mining and brainstorming during which Phil asked me the question: who do you respect the most in your life? We decided on a colleague and mentor of mine, George, a scholar and professor, who had in his life fought the guardians of Hades in the form of addiction and a lung disorder—and won. One night back in March, after I'd returned from Mom and Dad's, in the midst of the Tesla lunacy, this hound slayer and his wife had joined us for dinner, which had meant a day of Windex, micro-fiber dust cloths, the feather duster, and a commercial floor cleaner known for its ability to clean and wax floors simultaneously. I'll call it Slop and Shine.

Using Slop and Shine, as you might imagine, is not in keeping with our goal of biodegradable living. It is actually pretty funky, a chemical goo that cleans, disinfects, and polishes the kitchen floor all at once—like an automatic car wash in a bottle—and which is not supposed to be rinsed off. It is the lazy approach to floor care—or, better put, the harried, thank-goodness-they-make-such-a-product, young-wife-and-mother's approach to floor care. In my day, shining the floor required stripping it with ammonia first, rinsing several times, then spreading around your basic floor wax (we even had a long-handled appliance called a wax applicator to facilitate the job), which acted and smelled a little like liquid paraffin. It was effective, and lasted for weeks—months even, if the flow of traffic was as minimal as ours. But it takes time, and if it is not stripped away from time to time, it builds in yellowy layers, and those ammonia fumes aren't all that healthy either, so as I moved on to other things besides parenting and domesticity, I dispensed with the process in favor of your basic soap and water or, when I'm financially bulgy, one of those so-called green floor cleaners, which usually do not involve leaving a high-gloss finish. The older I get, however, for some reason I once again want my floors to reflect light. Maybe it is some brand of post-traumatic stress, but spending even fifteen minutes mopping a floor and ending with it only being clean is a disappointment. I want shine.

So it was that after my visit to Boise with Sean and Susannah for Leah's birth, and after mopping their kitchen floor with Slop and Shine and seeing the sock-skating results, the first thing I did after arriving back home was go to our local supermarket and buy the biggest bottle they sold. I didn't tell Phil what I had done or what product I had purchased, and the stuff still gets stored in the back of the under-the-sink kitchen cupboard where I know he never looks (because what man does?), but each time I mopped with it he commented on the great shine, and when he asked how I achieved it, I simply lied and said, "I waxed it." He surely must have caught on, but if he did, he never said anything. Meantime, I made sure to do the mopping chore when he wasn't around. I didn't exactly want him to know I was trading well-being for esthetics, nor did I want to endure the ribbing I'd receive for using such an environmentally unsound product. Besides, we were closer to being finished with our lives than we were to the beginning, although I was certain we both still had a very long way to go before meeting that final day, so perhaps the risk was excusable. By golly when I do go to the big Whatever-is-Next, at least I know I'll leave a pert and perky, glossy kitchen floor behind.

On my mind during the day's preparations for the evening's guests were happy endings. The week before George and his wife's visit we had Jacob, my youngest, and his more-gorgeous-than-ever-now-that-she's-pregnant wife Kelsey over for dinner. I had planned to prepare Eggplant Parmesan from *The Moosewood Cookbook* with a veal version for them. Son Jacob's response to my plan surprised me: "Do you know what they do to those poor calves? Lock them in a box from birth so that their meat stays pale and undeveloped. That's where the flavor and texture comes from." We decided on chicken instead, but never did I feel more self-righteous about choosing a vegetarian diet. I knew there was more than one reason, but I did not know this one, since I have never cared for veal. But all I could think of was our hobbling of free-spirited Tesla, whose photo captioned with his old name "Ernie" had begun appearing again in *The Lewiston Morning Tribune* classifieds.

Happy endings all around, it turned out. Jacob and Kelsey, their baby due October 11th, were about to purchase a house they'd wanted to buy for a while. Jacob's position at work was looking increasingly secure as time passed. He was the kid I worried about most. His childhood was very dramatic, since his father and I separated when he was seven and I subsequently did not get my feet under me until long after he had left the house and graduated college. It was ten-year-old Jacob that I picked up one day without warning from his fourth grade class and drove back to La Grande, where we had raised him, to live with his father. "Tough love," his counselors called it. At that time, he'd been behaving more and more like he had the makings of a juvenile delinquent, getting into fights, bloodying noses on the playground, breaking a child's arm in a tussle, vandalizing a school bus (oddly enough, at nineteen, he became the youngest bus driver in the history of one of our local school systems and drove his way through the last three years of his college career). Now a church-goer and a police officer, whether or not my antidote to his behavior worked is anyone's guess, but he did eventually come back to live with me during his high school years and stayed in the area for college and to raise his family. I was proud of the work he had done to overcome his anger and my machinations (my solution to any problem has always been to flee; he turns and faces the monster). I liken his journey to that of your average hero, who must face battle after battle before arriving at victory. No wonder he chose a degree in theater, and he can spout more literature than his university-English-instructor mother.

Also cause for cheer was the fact that my oldest son, Sean, had been offered a position. This after more than a year of unemployment after the start-up company he'd worked for folded in 2009. I'll save the details, since the CEO was involved in an international scandal and was the subject of news headlines for weeks, but I can sum it up by saying that Sean followed his instincts, suffered through a situation for no wages because he had a hunch it would in one way or another work out, and it did. Also in keeping with the hero's journey, rescue came at the last moment, just as he and Susannah were deciding they could no longer pay their mortgage on a house they had purchased new and moved into just months before he'd received his last full paycheck. When they headed back home after the wedding they would be heading into a new future, one with a significant pay raise and solid potential. No more start-ups for Sean. Unless things changed before the weekend, he was now part of the big-time.

If you believe TV stereotypes, lunch with a daughter-in-law is supposed to be fraught with jealous competition. Not so with Sean's wife, Susannah, who had become my ex-officio wedding planner and official photographer and who also at some point back earlier in the year had sat down with me to try to pull from my subconscious an image of what the setting for the wedding might look like. Thanks to her creative eye, by the end of lunch we had a theme flower (calla lilies) and secondary flowers (daylilies and stargazers). Perhaps she had stored in some nook in the back of her mind the fact that our rings were carved with lilies and doves, but I doubt it. I didn't remember it myself until I sat down to compose this paragraph. I much prefer to think she's simply connected with me beyond the realm of brains and memory and that the small, blue light of her purest self was able to discern lilies—associated with spirituality, purity of thought and action, abundance, friendship, and devotion—as representing the equally pure center of my relationship with Phil. Susannah's favorite, the pink stargazer, denotes immense wealth and prosperity, which I couldn't help but deem appropriate, given Sean's new employment status, and the immense wealth of family we all now shared.

And so our dining room had been for weeks a cathedral of flowers to be cleared before my colleague and his wife arrived for dinner. Susannah and I had made a haul of unexpectedly lovely silk lilies, looking more real than real; consequently, my dining table was a beast of burden laden with mimetic beauty. Phil claimed he could smell them when I walked in the front door with both arms full. Alas, it was only my hand sanitizer, but I knew what he meant. It seemed they should eventually begin to wilt, and it worried me every time I passed them. They were flanked by wands of calla lilies and two stacks of white rose garlands, one for the tables and one for head garlands for the three flower girls. Glass bud vases and cut glass mint dishes. A lovely cream-colored Victorian-style vase for the guest book table. On my way home I had stopped at a nursery to order fifty cut calla lilies and twenty-five stargazer lilies to flank the silk ones and truly generate that scent. Suddenly, I was Alice in Wedding Wonderland.

* * *

I suppose I should write about what it was like to be getting married for the third time, at the age of fifty-three. About how the largess—the loving partner, the beautiful Victorian—was not what I truly wanted for my life, although it was what my choices had indirectly created. Funny how I ached for so many years to escape what I saw as culture-less and soulless, the regions known as the Palouse, the Lewis-Clark Valley, and collectively part of the Intermountain West. But chose to stay because I wanted to remain near my children. For the first fifteen years I hated life in this place. Hated it. Despised it with sometimes intensity. I imagined myself belonging in some large city—Seattle, Chicago, New York—where people at the pinnacle of literature and art resided. How did I get to be someone who moved to the remote, rural American West for a two-year job on an Indian reservation and now it is twenty-two years later? The first twenty of which I spent trying to escape? And in that same now I was finding the place inspiring and beautiful and enlightening and bursting with interesting stories.

Perhaps it *was* the Vitamin D.

Phil said he began looking at the area on the map in the early 1990s, coincidentally just as I was lighting in Lewiston, separated from my husband and a single mother and lost.

The reason I was divorced the second time really came down to fitness. My second husband, to whom I was married for twelve years and who was the father of both Jacob and Sean, had hated the way I looked and hated the fact that clearly I would always have to work at being of a normal weight. He was a wild game and potatoes man; I, at odds with my genetics, which predisposed me to conserve calories in times of famine, lay down fat in times of plenty. My life's struggle.

My first marriage never should have occurred. It was just me, cloaked as a rebellious teenager, trying to get back at my parents for being the people they had been. The details don't matter, other than to say it was a classic example of an eighteen-year-old knowing a whole lot less than she thought she did. But it's worth mentioning that with my first husband, even though we were just homeless-last-of-the-hippies wandering and wondering around the country, my problems were the same: When I married I was of a normal weight; in the months immediately following the wedding, I got fat.

And, here I was again, except that now I was in my early fifties, with a body that had survived all the ups and downs, and about to marry a man who was okay with all that, but I felt so bad about the way I was going to look at the ceremony. And my dress size! An eighteen! First time, it had been a size eight, ditto the second time. Ugh! And I had adopted a habit of far less grooming over the years—less make-up, less fuss with the hair in terms of style and color. I prepared for our wedding day thinking that if we had simply stood alone before the county judge, I would not have to feel obsessed about my vaguely unkempt appearance. Writers are supposed to look vaguely unkempt. We couldn't care less about tanned skin, coiffed hair, and brand-name clothing. I had grown quite attached to physical inactivity, ponytails, and years-old, shapeless, un-ironed clothing.

Alas, we *were* having a public wedding, and I *did* care about how I was going to look next to Phil and our guests and in photographs. So, after visiting my parents and having and giving up a dog had caused me to temporarily embrace a food-and-couch addiction, I was now in better-get-on-the-stick mode, and frantically so. Daily, purposeful exercise and early evening gardening would do the trick. I hoped.

Conversation at Starbuck's one morning before the Alaska trip:

Me: "Any idea where to go for a wedding dress around here? For somebody old?"

Barista: "No. That's why I never got married."

Number of wedding shops in Lewiston and Clarkston: two.

Number of wedding dress Internet sites for Plus Sizes: maybe six.

Number of wedding dress possibilities after looking at more than 1,000 actual images of wedding-ish dresses: Zero.

Perfect film to watch when the world is making you feel like shit for the way you look: *Precious*.

* * *

And in the background, poor Phil. Two years prior he dug a hole in the ground for a pond. In the summer of 2009, he transformed a flower bed extending from the deck into another small pond. In March 2010, he sculpted a waterfall from turquoise quartz between the small pond and the big hole, outlining the big hole with the same rock. In early April, he had lined the big hole with carpet and a rubberized lining for backyard water features. On the day I went looking for a wedding dress for the first time, he filled everything with water and plugged in the pump. The pump worked just fine, if we were pumping punch from an ice sculpture. "All dressed up and no place to go," he said of the small dribble of water.

I hoped that was not the way we would feel once the wedding did come.

Despite the fact that Phil strangely enough didn't completely understand the physics of why a larger force moves more water through the same size hose than a smaller force, he finally relented and bought a more powerful pump for the pond. The result was a bona fide waterfall adding to the lyrical sounds of the friends and family who would be attending our wedding. By arranging his rock collection into the purchased sluice that constituted the smaller pond adjacent to the deck, the sound became that of a small creek, not unlike the many creeks next to which he and I had both camped in our separate lives, not unlike Petty's Fork Creek, which formed the boundary of my family's original Kentucky homestead.

*   *   *

Anyone who has not yet watched *Food, Inc.*, should do so before eating the next bite of chicken, hamburger, or meat of any kind. I was certainly surprised to learn that today there are only thirteen meatpacking firms in this country, whereas in the 1970s there were many thousands. The strain of E-coli that has killed so many evolved from feeding corn to cattle to fatten them. Cows are not meant to eat corn. In my family's part of the world, and in the south in general, where tobacco was once the ruling crop, farmers are raising chickens, mostly for Tyson Foods. Chickens are now engineered to grow from chick to slaughter in almost half the time and to twice their normal size with breasts so large they aren't even able to balance themselves to walk. We first saw this film late in 2009, and after seeing it again on PBS in the weeks just prior to the wedding, I remembered that *Food, Inc.*, and two other films we had seen that autumn, *The Future of Food* and *Two Angry Moms*, were what first influenced me toward returning to vegetarianism. I was so glad for that decision. I would never have had the energy to create a wedding celebration otherwise.

And there we were, with mere weeks to go, impeded by rain with more predicted. All my weeding? For naught. Except that the new ones taking their place were only four inches high. Had I not weeded, they'd likely reach mid-calf. I wished I had a nice, big cow to chew them down, but I feared she would not be selective and would take out the vinca, the lilies, the tulips, the lavender, the sage, the columbine, the oat grass, the succulents, the astragalus, the peonies, the pansies, the ranunculus, the mint, the asters, the rosemary, the roses, the hyacinths, the chives, the lilacs, the begonias, and the daisy starts as well.

Meanwhile, money marched from our wallets and much faster and in bigger chunks than it had when we'd acquired Tesla: cake, cut flowers, more plant life for the gardens.

Finally, however, Phil's backyard sculptures were nearly complete, and in their completeness were total opposites of each other. The rock garden looked more like a glacial deposit, so natural was its shape and appearance. The Spanish lavender and rosemary could have been mistaken for sage, so long as you didn't get too close. Chocolate mint likes to stay wet, we had found, so it was plucked from its aridity-loving neighbors and stationed in a pot within easy watering reach of the deck as we did all but mouth-to-mouth to try and resuscitate it, and an overdose of H_2O turned out to be all that was needed. The waterfall and pond, framed and outlined in angular turquoise quartz, stood in stark juxtaposition to the rock garden's smooth-stoned river granite. Surely those two were spawned from the same process, since they were indigenous to our area, but you'd never have known it to look at them. One featured the clawing scramble of cliff work, the other the grace and tumble of time and water wear. One a deposit, one an erosion. Both the product of fire and pressure.

Inside, thanks to the rain impeding outdoor work, we were reminded that nothing improves the vibrations of a home like a good, solid cleaning. Windex, dish soap for the blinds, and Murphy's Oil Soap were my friends in those waning days. What no one tells you is that at fifty, every fiber of your body launches itself onto a life of its own. These independent components are lazy bastards who bellyache and complain every time you insist on engaging them, even if it is for their own good. This painful noise is accentuated one hundred-fold for every year beyond fifty, especially when they are forced to do housework.

The rainy evenings gave me time to hunt for more dresses-for-the-voluptuous websites, and one night I finally found the perfect dress in which to be married a third and, hopefully, final time. My other two weddings featured dresses I sewed myself: the first a quasi-traditional, Juliet silhouette made of a somewhat expensive slinky, shiny, knit fabric called Qiana, and with a train and lace accents; the second a hippie-ish, gauze skirt and balloon-sleeved blouse in flocked batiste. Both in ivory, both uniquely my style, both lovely to me.

And so I faced the truth of the measuring tape. For all the hemp shakes, meatless meals, general abstaining, random exercising, forced marches, endless planting, weeding, and myriad activity planning the wedding had required, to purchase a "designer" dress meant to be lumped back into my previous size range: "Plus-size customers, please note, our designer fashions are known to run smaller than off-the-rack." And a size eighteen was considered plus-size.

Bah. Humbug.

* * *

And then, finally, the short-notice trip to Alaska to do a bit of consulting work and earn a bit of extra cash for the honeymoon, which ended with me inhaling a broncho-dilator for weeks and weeks to come and wishing there were a way to mainline mullein.

I cannot reveal why I had to fly into the Alaskan tundra three weeks before my May twenty-second wedding because, on a very part-time basis, I am a federal sub-contractor and have signed an agreement stating that I will not discuss the details of what I do, except that it has to do with helping people.

But I can tell you what it is like to crawl into a bush plane and to be flown across miles and miles of earth melting at its varying spring paces, its color morphing from wedding white to shades of coffee and cream. To have been able to survey the earth where it is flattened, the sky broadened and marginless. To have at my forebrain the life and memories of Beryl Markham from my 2009 reading of *West With the Night* and now to understand why humans so crave flight, to wonder if my vegetarian diet will render me thin enough that I can walk to an aviation school counter, hand over my hard-won dollars and say, "Teach me to fly."

I can tell you what it is to have the gleeful little girl in me restored and squealing from being bundled in the bed of a blue, handmade wooden sled, popping across the tundra at the whims of a Yupik man and his Ski-doo with its Frankenstein conglomeration of skis and caterpillar traction, wondering if my federal status was enough to make him want to drop me into parts from which I might never return.

And I can tell you what it is to spend a day and a night in a village of indigenous people who for some reason are comfortable living in a place hundreds of impassible miles from any other humans, where their homes are built on stilts, and which are connected by a constellation of board sidewalks, because at certain parts of the year, to venture otherwise is to sink into the very earth the rest of us trust so unconsciously to hold us. And I can tell you what it is to wish I never had to leave again, because for the first time in my life, despite the hundreds of days and miles I have ventured into the mountains and forests of the

Pacific Northwest, I now knew what it was to breath clean air and feel my home planet at its purest.

And, I can tell you about an extra little miracle.

The morning I was to fly out of Lewiston and Clarkston, my plane, a brand new plane, was inexplicably grounded. Inexplicably because the plane's computer flashed an engine warning light, but no mechanic could find a problem. They flew in a man from Pullman: he couldn't find it. They were flying a man in from Seattle; that would take more time. The next thing we knew we were being reorganized onto other flights. Mine would require waiting in Seattle. *Seven and a half hours*. I would not arrive in Anchorage until almost midnight. I would start the trip tired, because who can sleep when they go to bed at midnight knowing they have to get up at four a.m. to catch a flight into the Alaskan tundra? And then continue the trip tired because I would not reach my second hotel room until after one a.m. the *next* day, knowing I would have to leave for the airport yet again another four hours later. A friend and former colleague at WSU, who was the only person I knew in Seattle, was kind enough to pick me up at the Seattle airport and say, "We are finding your dress."

To Southcenter Mall, to Nordstrom Rack, then the dressbarn. We were in the dressbarn fewer than ten minutes when I found it— them, to be accurate. I turned a corner, walked to the rack, and picked up the two items that were to become my wedding attire. The off-shoulder top and black skirt sparkled. They swirled. They draped from my shoulders and hips in an array that said, "Twenty pounds— gone!" even when it was hard to detect considering how heavy I was to begin with. With the new haircut done in an updo, the new color weave, I should easily pass as the star of the show. I wondered how it would feel, looking at Phil standing there waiting for me, knowing all we know and the way we've lived these past three and a half years. If the tarot reading I'd recently consulted was any indication, I would feel like I was home.

Elemental changes. That is what I told those close to me before I left for Alaska: "I feel like this trip is going to change me in some elemental way." I did not know that meant I would develop a severe allergic reaction to toxic black mold that would turn my lungs into amphibian gills and leave me airless and voiceless for nearly two months—grave, systemic symptoms, the after-effects of which would still haunt me three years later.

I dealt with it by swallowing massive doses of mullein tincture, all the while sucking periodically on a Proventil inhaler, the prescription for which Phil managed to obtain from a physician. I was willing to partake of that scientific/chemical product because I knew what I probably needed was a night or two in the hospital and systemic Diflucan to kill that inhaled black mold. Things were bad. But I believed my condition could resolve itself if I could give my body the right support, and I knew one of mullein's many properties was as an antifungal. I needed that inhaler because I simply didn't have time to lie down and recuperate, and Phil does usually have a rescue inhaler on hand. It wasn't too far off the mark to call his physician and say he was having seasonal allergies, take in his expired inhaler, and get a new one.

Had I known then what I know now, I would have recognized my body's dramatic warning and reorganized the month of May 2010, so that it did not include a wedding. Fortunately—or unfortunately, depending on at which point during the ensuing two years you were to ask me—being a twenty-first century American, and as we've already established, I am not overly intuitive.

As it was, I returned from that Alaska trip gripped with fever and preoccupied myself with the hope that sixty thousand biodegradable rose petals would be enough to cover the yard's grassless places. We were down to thinking about those sorts of details.

Food, of course, was top-of-the-list, too. Early on, we found ourselves quarreling with whether to impose our new habits on our guests, opted instead to include a barbecued brisket and pulled pork alongside my vegetarian lasagna. Neither of us would be tempted. But we discussed whether our coastal honeymoon would feature a seafood dish or two. Even if seafood is perhaps the most contaminated of our food sources, fresh grilled oysters on the half-shell are little rocky cups of heaven, as far as my perspective is concerned, and I may like them even better deep fried. Just in case, we were packing a bottle of papaya enzyme for the honeymoon. The body is efficient enough in its operations that it only manufactures what enzymes it needs: if you eat beans, it generates bean enzymes; if you eat the flesh of living beings, it generates living-being enzymes. Not tossing back a papaya enzyme capsule or two before consuming meat or seafood in the wake of a plant-based diet will result in joint pain and swelling. If this sounds like the voice of experience, it is. I remember having to eat bottles of the stuff when dysbiosis required me to transition back to a meat-based diet in the mid-90s. Would I feel I had reneged on my promises to health, my body, and the planet if I ate those grilled oysters? Not on your life. Naughtiness at times is necessary. Oysters on a honeymoon are a giggly prerequisite—wink wink—worth whatever shame, whatever risk.

Meantime I prayed nightly to the Goddess of Blooming: make the chestnut and hawthorn blossoms stay just as they are for a few more days. I promised I would never again complain about the Yeti-sized bumblebees their aromatic flowers attracted. Or the holes in the flower beds the squirrels dug to store their nutty harvest for winter feasts.

Despite the severity of my illness, and amidst interviews on the phone with my contracting agency to describe the circumstances around my exposure to toxic black mold, explain the progression, and describe the reasons for self-treatment of my symptoms, wedding preparations continued, and the bits of magic. Such as gallon-sized maidenhair ferns for ten dollars and ninety-seven cents each. They were more like bushes. Which I found one morning after saying to Phil, "I'd love to have a couple of ferns on either side of that waterfall." I knew they were mispriced. They should have been twenty-one dollars and ninety-seven cents like all the other gallon-sized plants next to them. Maybe to take them was a sin and would bring bad luck, but I didn't care. Twenty-one dollars and ninety-seven cents each wasn't in the budget. I felt like the error was a blessing, a gift from God. Then there were the adorable Japanese paper lanterns from the Dollar Store for a dollar each, in vibrant hues of the faded strawberry, pale lemon, and pale aqua, colors we had chosen to dominate the wedding palette, plus AAA batteries, each lamp requiring two, also a buck. And then demure, cannellated-crystal champagne glasses from Pier One for seven dollars each. Perfectly weightless and perfect for us. Then the even more magical floating candles. Shapes of faded strawberry and pale lemon flowers and green leaves, eight for three dollars. Masculine fire met feminine water, in the old marriage tradition, in the form of these floating flames. We planned to light them and lower them into the pond after the cake was eaten and my calla lily bouquet thrown. Phil's nephew was to be responsible for replacing melted candles with new ones, until the guests had gone home.

The days of work ticked, and the rain fell. We sat by the pond late at night and listened to the waterfall. It was loud and soft as a creek. Still so much to do. We had not finished painting the kitchen cabinets. Even though guests would not be indoors, we had plenty of family who would, and some of the male factions of the bridal party were to be staying in the house. We just couldn't let them be privy to our partially painted cupboards. Plus, Phil hadn't found a suit. I hadn't found shoes. And I wanted so badly to paint my sunburst—a large architectural feature yard-sale find I'd owned for more than a decade and which we had situated on the east side of the yard to mimic the rising sun and to symbolize our new beginnings—a beautiful morning yellow, but moisture kept coming, and we did not have indoor space large enough to do it.

WANING GIBBOUS MOON

I DON'T KNOW HOW I WOULD HAVE MADE IT that day if it were not for my daughter-in-law, Susannah, who is not only the mother of my two oldest granddaughters, but also a fabulously talented photographer of people and who was the official photographer for the wedding. I keep telling her she is an artist. That she has a gift. Under her guidance, cajoling, and effervescence, we all looked like celebrities.

And then my other daughter-in-law, Kelsey, radiant, generous, and infinitely caring, gracefully moved through the day with my first grandson just starting to produce a visible round in her profile, doing errand after errand the morning of the wedding, when I called for rescue at eight a.m. because no one in the household, save Phil and I, was out of bed. She also spent the day serving admirably as Susannah's assistant.

Despite all the amazing help I had that day, I also have to give a dab of credit to my dress. Every woman reading this knows how much confidence can come from the right dress, no matter what the situation.

As I've mentioned, it was a skirt and blouse. Beaded buttermilk chiffon over a silk jersey tank top lining, with cutwork sleeves and hem and a draping, almost-off-the-shoulder neckline. The bead- and cutwork, in the shape of lilies, echoed the lilies carved into the polished silver of our rings, and those gracing the podium, the serving tables, the dinner tables, Phil's sisters' corsages, the bouquet I carried, and the single-stem calla lily each of the women of the bridal court held. The black chiffon gored skirt flowed and swirled just right, and my colleague from Seattle who had helped me find my dress had surprised me with a gift she crafted herself—onyx and freshwater pearl earrings and bracelet that perfectly tied the two pieces together. "You get to be a princess, too, G-ma?" my granddaughter Malory said.

The day, even still, does not come as one linear memory, but a foggy pastiche. I was sick on the day of my third wedding, and that pretty much says it all. I'm not the first bride to go through it, I'm certain, but I wish it had been otherwise. I wanted so to enjoy that day with Phil. My other two weddings had been special in their own way, but I married those two people for ridiculous reasons. I was marrying Phil because I enjoyed him. I enjoyed living with him, and he seemed to reciprocate. We were a reflection of each other, and that is what we romantic humans all wish for. I'm not so naïve as to believe that "one true love" exists for each and every one of us nearly seven billion people on this planet, but for almost seven years of coupledom now, I have consistently marveled at how much we have in common, just the same as I was marveling then.

Occasional moments do stand out, however. For example, seeing my two strong, capable, handsome sons, Sean and Jacob, in suits and ties and having them tell me how beautiful I looked as they took their places on either side of me for the ceremony, our arms linked. Jacob had called my parents and lent his cell phone so that Mom and Dad, too frail to travel, could be witness to the ceremony. How I loved in that moment the feeling of being cared for and supported by those two wonderful people. In one way or another it's always been Sean and Jacob shoring me up, giving me reason to be.

Phil's two great-nieces Tara and Nathalie served alongside Malory as the most adorable flower girls in history. I had sent snippets of strawberry, lemon, and aqua ribbon and just asked their mothers to pick dresses that matched and that the girls might wear later, so they were each in dresses of different design and color, yet their little flower crowns with ribbon veils were the same. Nothing inspires more joy or is more memorable than a flower girl at a wedding.

One of the funnier moments came when my good friend Jill Nugent was referred to as "some strange woman in the driveway." She and I still laugh about it. We should all be brave enough to wear dreadlocks at fifty-something, and we should all be brave enough to do the work she does in Haiti, teaching people to plant community gardens, teaching them how to improve their meager lives, bringing back the grace and wisdom that permeates their most difficult of situations.

I remember Fred, the retired Lutheran pastor we finally found who was willing to do the legal work and let my colleague George do the poetic stuff, putting on his Elmer Fudd hat when the wind picked up during the reception and the weather turned chilly.

I remember how insanely, moan-worthy good our wedding cake was. I mean the best, best cake you could ever *not* come even close to imagining was possible. It was a perfectly lemony, exceptionally creamy, meltaway-textured yellow iced lemon chiffon we ordered from our favorite artisan bakery. They don't usually make wedding cakes, but we talked them into taking three of their lemon chiffon cakes, which normally come in a brick shape, and stacking them one on two to make them look like a single entity. They did, and it was an unusual and stunning work of art, and that moment is studded into my brain's memory lobe forever, all those wedding guests swooning in ecstasy after the first bite and having each of those people ask, "Who did this cake?" and hearing, over and over again, "This is the best cake I've ever eaten!"

And I remember being stunned by the fact that my friend Kathy had saved rose petals for an entire month to be tossed and strewn along with my sixty thousand "silk" ones from the Dollar Store.

And I remember the food.

Phil's sisters had managed the kitchen and the reception for us, but Phil and I did a great deal of the cooking ourselves. We made Lasagna Al Forno for the main dish, which disappeared before I could get any, but also had that brisket specially fire-roasted for our omnivorous guests, plus Phil's award winning (literally—he has a plaque!) pulled pork, accompanied by his Famous Baked Beans—a vegetarianized version of his sister's recipe. Among other well-received dishes, both vegetarian and omnivore, was my mother's time-worn recipe for potato salad. We prefer the skins on, but Mom would never hear of it. She always slipped them off. My rule is, if you use organic potatoes, keep the skins. Also, don't substitute organic mayo. The taste just isn't the same. And make sure you cook and chop the potatoes, eggs, and onion exactly as specified, else the flavor and texture won't be exact, either.

Kentucky Potato Salad for a Crowd

10 pounds large russet potatoes
1 dozen eggs
2 large yellow onions, finely chopped
1 16-ounce jar sweet pickle relish
Best Foods Mayonnaise
Prepared mustard (we use Natural Value Organic)
Sea salt
Fresh ground black pepper
Paprika

Boil potatoes until they just barely yield to a fork. Do not overcook. Turn off heat, cover pan, and let potatoes sit in water until it is completely cool. In the meantime, place eggs in a pot, cover with water, and bring to a boil. Remove from heat and let sit until water is cool. In a very large bowl, quarter potatoes lengthwise and then quarter again horizontally. Chop eggs into 1/2-inch cubes and add to bowl with potatoes. Add onion and relish. Mix. Stir in 1 cup mayo then add 1 tablespoon at a time and stir until mixture is slightly creamy. Stir in 1 tablespoon mustard then add more and mix to taste. Add salt and black pepper to taste. Garnish liberally with paprika. Cover and refrigerate overnight before serving.

Phil's Famous Baked Beans

1 14-ounce can vegetarian "pork" and beans
1 14-ounce can white beans
1 14-ounce can kidney beans
1 14-ounce can black beans
1 onion, chopped
1/4 cup coconut sugar
1/4 cup ketchup
Cayenne pepper
Italian seasoning
Garlic powder

Preheat oven to 275 degrees. Mix first seven ingredients in an oven-safe casserole dish. Add seasonings to taste. Slow bake uncovered for 45 minutes. Serves 8.

*　*　*

Remaining vegetarian on our road-trip honeymoon, which we had vowed to do our best to enjoy despite how ill I remained, required diligence. As a result, we were occasionally sideswiped by things like bacon in a fabulous gourmet breakfast sandwich at The Olive in Walla Walla, Washington. Innocent mistake. We thought those little chunks were red onions and that it was simply the best breakfast sandwich either of us had ever eaten. The night before it was gnocchi cooked in chicken broth on what was advertised as a vegetarian dish. We were hungry enough in Burns, Oregon, to pretend the beef broth in the Thai noodles was soy sauce. Our other choices for dinner that particular evening were slim and involved pizza made on pre-fab crusts in a family-frenzied locally owned pizzeria. We shored ourselves with enough boiled eggs to last the week once we made it to the beach house in Oceanside, Oregon, pun intended. Vegetable pâtè, hummus, and canned dolmas in the road-trip goody bag packed for us by a friend got us through a slim evening when neither of us felt hungry until the only restaurant in Oceanside was already closed.

But a few places were obviously accustomed to serving vegetarian patrons and were doing it well. The Deschutes Brewery made a delectable bean burger, and we breakfasted twice at Bend Mountain Coffee, enjoying something called Umpqua Oats, which was more like trail mix than morning fare, and which we loved so much, even though Phil normally doesn't care for oats, that we bought four of their little carton/bowls to take with us and planned to order a case just as soon as the dust from a year of wedding planning settled. The coffee was undeniably the most soulful and rich either of us had tasted in quite some time. Starbucks lost me in favor of Strictly Organic Coffee Company's Organic Sustainability Blend. The Green Salmon in coastal Yachats made fruit juice-sweetened morning scones so chock full of oats you couldn't get through a whole one, no matter how badly you wanted to, so filling were they. Between Umpqua Oats and those scones, our personal cholesterol levels surely dropped a dozen points. But the prize went to Heidi's, also in Yachats, where the handmade vegetarian lasagna and four-cheese ravioli were the best restaurant Italian dishes either of us could remember, surpassed only by their apple pie with amaretto sauce. My shining example of perfect apple pie has always been from the kitchen of a man named Harv in St. Maries, Idaho, who could take a bagful of Granny Smiths, a handful of sugar, and a bit of cinnamon, throw them into a pie crust, and an hour or so later set you up with your own belt-ripping slice of dessert heaven. He had a secret to both the crust and the filling he refused to share, no matter how stern and eternal the interrogation. I suspected from the flavor it was a dash of whiskey, even though he swore himself to be a teetotaler. But he was always happy to stir up his deep-dish version for company and for bake sales, every bite always the same: apples tasting like pure green late summer, never sweet enough to notice but sweet enough to make apple juice stand up and shout. You could balance that sweetness on your tongue like a scale; it would never tilt one way or another. The crust was, as all good pie crusts are, made with lard, thin as a razor on top, a few slivers thicker on the bottom, crimped together with a fork, painted with milk, sprinkled with sugar, and baked golden. Heidi's pie was Harv's pie gone delirious. The crust was just that much thicker and flakier, the apples baked to butter-firm, noticeably unnoticeably sweet, but then there was that pale, dreamy, organic sugar-butter sauce laced with amaretto. Forget the ice cream. With this pie, all you had to do was light a candle, say a prayer for the self you were leaving behind, and dig in, taking slow, slow, slow measured bites, each chew in equally-paced, movie-show slow-mo, the mastication now initiating the body's chemical processes wherein each hollowed, trembling forkful begins melting into your cellular structure, finally reaching that last-bit-of-crust moment when you lapse, eyes closed, into a sparkling, mystic, psychic comma of a coma, the Red Sea parting of your earthly existence. That is to say, it ran a close second to our wedding cake.

An undetermined amount of time later, shaken awake by the waiter's question of "How was it?" I returned to the planet emboldened by the knowledge that I was emerging a changed human. Endorphins rushed through my body. Colors in the room were heightened and bright. I felt my cheeks flush with health and well-being, my pulse slowed to a rare-for-me meditative rate. I was a living Zen moment. I declared the pie, "Best Ever," in a throaty whisper, coughed to clear my voice and take control of myself again, once more proclaiming— and more definitively—"This is, hands down, the best piece of pie I've ever eaten." And I said this in unison with my new husband, who'd obviously just had the same experience and who I swear was surrounded by a faint, sunny aura, inhabiting his own altered plane of existence. I think it was a moment of deep remembering—after a year of dog anxiety and house overhaul and wedding planning—of what was at our core: a love of well-prepared food.

At Heidi's, it turns out, if a patron mentions the words, "Best Ever," he or she is urged to comment in their "Best Ever" journal. And so it was that my written assessment of The Best Apple Pie Ever lives *in memoriam* to attest to that fact.

* * *

And then the rain. Days and nights and nights and days of endless rain. If Noah had been tent camping when the floods started, he'd have drowned. We had decided to end the circle of our road-trip "weddingmoon" as we came to call it, with camping on The Lochsa River, which is, if such a thing is possible, my "soul's river." It is a place—as someone once termed it—where my "insides match my outside." The Lochsa runs east to west, separating the Idaho Panhandle from the bulk of the state. It is formed by the confluence of Crooked Fork and Colt Killed Creeks and joins with the Selway River seventy miles west to form the Clearwater, which flows into the Snake River at the mouth of Hell's Canyon, North America's deepest gorge, near the Lewis-Clark Valley where we live. I love the dramatic changes, the way every spring snowmelt re-sculpts the Lochsa's banks. At the time of our trip, it was an unseasonable excess of rain following a late snow dump and quick melt. We camped, or tried to camp, at Powell Campground, at milepost 162, near the Powell Ranger Station and the Lochsa Lodge, an historic stopover twenty miles to the east over the Continental Divide from the well-known Lolo Hot Springs. Suffice it to say, we repeatedly drove the pickup over the Rockies to soak the cold from our bones in the hot springs and more than once cold-footed it to the lodge, a short hike from the campground, where we could pay someone to cook for us, rather than stand shivering over the Coleman lit only for the heat, eating meals of cheese and crackers because it was just too dang cold to do anything else.

Phil's job required him to be in Big Hole, Montana, on Tuesday, so the camping was a honeymoon bonus tag. After a day home to regroup we had headed east, pitched camp, and battled the weather. Big Hole is the site of the U.S. Army's famed pre-dawn attack on the band of Nez Perce Indians fleeing the government in 1877. Dozens of the aged, the infirm, women, and children were slaughtered in their sleep. While Phil presided over a meeting with a group of federal contractors, I hiked the trails through the Nez Perce camp and the battleground. The silence of the place had kept me awake the night before. Every time I dozed, I fell into dreaming of the listless wandering of the spirits of those Nez Perce men and women. I heard the moans of bludgeoned children. Smelled powder from rifle shots. Felt screams rip through my own living body, heart and brain trembling, rattled by the chaos of the battle that came to life around me. Whatever meager pains and disappointments existed in my little life became whispers in their presence. The next morning I sat in the midst of a grouping of skeletal tipis and paid homage to the benevolent forces of the universe asking them to forgive my human failures, send sustenance to those who needed it. "You are entering Sacred Ground," the government sign read. All ground is Sacred Ground, I wanted to argue, wondering why it is so often that human pain and suffering are what lead us to revere a place as sacred. Otherwise, all ground—our Mother Earth, the rivers and the rain that keeps them flowing—is simply holy. I held out my hand to catch the falling drops to soak in their blessings, thankful for the Sacred Ground of my and Phil's home, to which we were both starting to feel ready to return and to face the river-sized question—would this marriage outlast all our other ones? A year from now, would we be looking at a battleground? Would we cry ourselves to sleep at night? Would we bake bread together? Drink tea in the mornings? Never cheat?

* * *

We did discover one wondrous thing on the Lochsa trip: percolated coffee. Susannah's mother, Gwen, gave us the previous Christmas a stovetop percolator for camping. An old-fashioned gizmo for making coffee that involves putting ground coffee into a metal drip basket with a flat, metal top with perforations to also allow dripping. A tube passes from the bottom of the pot up through the filter and spurts boiling water, which falls atop the filter basket and drips through the grounds. You can see the water hit the lid top through its glass knob. As the circulated water turns brown, you lower the heat to the point that only one percolation occurs every two seconds. This was easily accomplished on our Coleman camp stove, but was trickier on the electric range in the park housing we stayed in at Big Hole, which responded slowly to changes in the thermostat. The beverage's strength is determined by how long the coffee is allowed to percolate at this rate. We quickly found that Starbucks French Roast needed very little time, no more than five minutes, but Strictly Organic Coffee Company's Organic Sustainability Blend loved to luxuriate. We left that perking for ten minutes and longer. Alas, by the end of the trip, the pound we bought in Bend was gone, but Starbucks French Roast was stunningly soulful, if smoky, if we didn't cook it too long, and was a welcome substitute. I have never liked machine-dripped coffee. As a result, for the last fifteen years or so, I've used either a single-cup filter (a Starbucks Gold Filter; it makes a near-perfect cup as well, and mine is as good as the day I bought it, even with daily use) or a French press. I'm always more or less in search of the perfect bean and roast cooked up in just the right way. The kitchen staff at the school in one of the Alaska villages I visited surprised me with an attention-getting cup of plain old Folgers, made in a similar stovetop percolator. It tasted so good I didn't even mind the Coffee-mate.

After our first taste of that first morning cup in the rain on the Lochsa, Phil and I both declared this stovetop percolated method as now part of our lives. It made us forget our troubles. But don't mistake this for your mother's electric percolator coffee. It is not the same. The water has to be boiling. And boiling takes fire. In fact, it's best to start with ice-cold spring water, just like my grandmothers used to do. I remember the sound of my dad's mother, Grandma Hazel, heading out to get water for coffee in the morning. The tin pail rattling against the door as she opened it. The decrescendo and crescendo of her leaving and returning footsteps, audible even on dew-damp grass. Then, once she was back in the house, the sound of the grounds going into the pot. The smell of it brewing as Grandpa came back from milking. People took their coffee with the cream off the top of fresh-from-the-cow milk, poured the first sips in their saucers to cool, and sipped from that until what was left in the cup was the optimum temperature to drink. In a right world, I start my coffee with refrigerated bottled spring water and top the finished product with organic half-and-half. It's as close to my grandmother's way as I can get unless I move to acreage and buy a cow, which I'm not apt to do. The coffee's depth and presence is communication from the bean, expressing appreciation for being well prepared.

* * *

One of the disadvantages of having spoiled ourselves on our honeymoon with good food wherever we could find it was that restaurant choices in the Lewis-Clark Valley once we returned home seemed doubly bleak in comparison. For some reason, that first night back, both our minds drifted to burritos and between the two of us we came up with a format that made even our eyeballs sweat.

Red-Hot, Four-Star, Two-Bean Burritos

1 15-ounce can pinto beans
1 15-ounce can black beans
1 tablespoon sunflower oil
1 tablespoon butter
sea salt to taste
1 cup cooked white organic basmati rice
2 tablespoons extra virgin olive oil
1/2 large green pepper, finely chopped
1/2 red onion, finely chopped
6 cloves garlic, minced

1/2 teaspoon ground cumin
1/4 teaspoon (or to taste) ground red chilis
1/8 teaspoon celery salt
1/4 cup plain tomato sauce
2 cups cold, filtered or spring water
Don Pancho's Gorditas Flour Tortillas
Tillamook Hot Habanero Jack Cheese, shredded
Nancy's Plain Lowfat Yogurt
Green chili sauce
1 small jicama, diced
1 avocado, diced

Beans:

Drain beans. Heat sunflower oil in a frying pan over a medium flame. Add butter and allow to melt. Add beans. Mash beans with fork or potato masher and add salt to taste. Fry until beans are heated thoroughly and dry. Cover and set aside.

Rice:

Heat olive oil in a frying pan over medium heat. Add green pepper, onion, and garlic. Sauté until onion is clear. Add cooked rice, cumin, ground chilies, and celery salt, stirring constantly until rice starts to brown. Add tomato sauce and stir until heated through. Add water. Heat over medium heat to boiling. Set heat to lowest setting and cover. Check at 20 minutes. Cook until rice flakes apart with a fork.

Burrito:

Set oven to 425 degrees. Preheat pizza stone. Warm tortillas one at a time on stone. Layer with beans, rice, cheese, yogurt, chili sauce, jicama, and avocado. Roll burrito-fashion and have a glass of milk close by when eating.

* * *

I embraced the knowledge that creating with food was a useful way to normalize emotions and keep ourselves rolling forward. I was still struggling with the effects of having inhaled toxic mold, but once back home and alone, we began to mine ourselves for old pre-dog, pre-wedding ways of being, and quickly found them. Phil's brunch dish our first weekend morning back was not new to either of us, but it was the first time he'd made it while I recorded it in recipe form. We were reminded of it during an overnight with his friends Tom and Ruth in Victor, Montana, following our stay at Big Hole. Ruth had made a similar version for us for brunch the last day of our three weeks on the road.

Brunch Florentine

3-4 slices 1/2-inch-thick sourdough bread*
8 eggs, beaten
3 cloves garlic, minced
1/2 teaspoon Tony Chachere's Original Creole Seasoning
2 cups baby spinach, washed and chopped
1/4 cup green chili sauce
1/4 cup half and half
1/4 cup whole milk
2 cups Tillamook Vintage White Extra Sharp Cheddar
        Cheese, shredded

Arrange bread in buttered 9x13 baking dish. Mix all other ingredients except cheese and pour over bread. Top with shredded cheese. Cover and let sit in refrigerator overnight. Bake the next morning at 350 degrees for 45 minutes. Allow to rest 15 minutes after removing from oven. Serve with minted fruit salad.

* Bread must be substantial rustic or artisan-type bread and should be several days old, not fresh. Grocery-store bread will dissolve.

*   *   *

The year progressed and eventually enough days passed that summer began showing signs of peaking—what summer we had in 2010, since the cool weather of spring was really what continued to drag us through the calendar. Still, by July, the yucca were in full bloom, the various strains of lilies, the lavender. I knew we'd tipped the seasonal scale when the lavender was ready to harvest. The other evidence was the blooming of the local farmer's market, where on Saturdays we picked up onions, pint jars of homemade strawberry-rhubarb jam, eggs, chard, and baby beets. An acquaintance of ours from Ghana who sells his family's basketry at local arts fairs had his booth set up, and when he learned Phil and I had married, gave us a lovely leather-handled market basket woven from plain and dyed grasses in which to transport our wares. The man once told me his father had had twenty wives, and they all made baskets. Basket weaving was a tradition also in my Kentucky mountain family, albeit we used hickory splints and twigs instead of the grasses of the Ghanan baskets. I attributed it to genetic impulses when, several decades ago, I began weaving egg baskets. I gave most of them away, but two still sat filled with dried flowers and trinkets in our guestroom downstairs. Not one of them had ever held an egg or jangled from an arm in a henhouse. I wondered how many of our friend's baskets got used for their original purposes.

The summer heat had Phil and I both struggling once again with low blood sugars: too hot to cook; too hot to eat. To the rescue, a large pot of Five Beans, some to freeze, some to mash into Five-Bean Sandwich Spread, some to store in the fridge for protein emergencies, and a double batch of Chard Summer Soup, served cold, and thankfully so. A cup of Five Beans whipped in the food processor with a jalapeno and a handful of cilantro made a great dip for Kirkland's Organic Tortilla Chips from Costco.

Five Beans

1 cup each dried kidney beans, navy beans, black beans, small
   red beans, and yellow lentils
1 large yellow onion, chopped
1 head garlic, peeled and minced

Rinse beans and lentils and place in large stew pot. Cover
with water and bring to boil. Turn off heat and let sit 1
hour. Add onion, garlic, and enough water that the liquid
over the beans is several inches deep. Simmer on low 1-
2 hours or until beans are soft. Divide and store in
freezer or refrigerator. Makes 5-6 quarts.

Five-Bean Sandwich Spread

1 cup Five Beans, drained, chilled, and mashed
1 hard-boiled egg, chopped
1/4 cup chopped green pepper
2 tablespoons capers
2 tablespoons pimentos
2 tablespoons sweet pickle relish
1 teaspoon orange zest
1+ tablespoons mayonnaise
Salt and fresh ground black pepper to taste
Dark rye bread
Butter lettuce
Yellow tomato slices
Provolone slices

Mix Five Beans, egg, green pepper, capers, pimentos, relish,
and orange zest, adding enough mayo to moisten mixture.
Season with salt and pepper. Spoon onto dark rye bread.
Dress with butter lettuce, tomato, and a slice of provolone.
Makes two hearty sandwiches.

Chard Summer Soup

3 tablespoons butter
3 tablespoons flour
3 cups vegetable broth
1 green tomato, very finely chopped
1 leek, very finely sliced
2 bunches chard, chopped
1/4 cup chopped mint plus more for garnish
4 strawberries, sliced

Make a roux with butter and flour over medium-low heat. Add broth, stirring in a bit at a time to avoid lumps. Add vegetables and mint. Cook over low heat until vegetables are very soft, adding small amounts of water as needed to keep mixture thinned. Remove from heat and allow to cool. Puree in blender. Garnish with mint leaves and strawberry slices. Serve cold. If green tomatoes are not available, tomatillos make an acceptable substitute. Serves 2.

FULL MOON AGAIN

SORTING THROUGH FILES BRINGS ME a certain peace of mind (one of the many things I did to try to heal myself of my illness from toxic mold and recover from the exhaustion of the wedding preparations and the school year and the Tesla drama was to slow way down and focus on doing small, quiet things) and often turns up forgotten gems, especially after thirteen years of teaching university English. Purging is always part of psychic recovery for me, figuratively relieving my system of weighted things, which can work against you like poison when you are struggling to enter a new phase of existence. The effect of the purging was not unlike Tesla chewing daffodils and grass. I came across this list from September 2000, that was forwarded to me by an instructor at Florida State University. No other credit was given as it was one of those ubiquitous emails which, on occasion, recirculate.

The Meaning of Love

Throughout the ages, our greatest writers and philosophers have wrestled with the problem of capturing in words the true essence of love. Children don't have nearly so much difficulty. In a recent survey, four- to eight-year-old children were happy to share their views on the subject. But what do little kids know about love? Read on and realize that kids already have a simple but deep grasp on that four-letter word.

- Love is that first feeling you feel before all the bad stuff gets in the way.

- When my grandmother got arthritis, she couldn't bend over and paint her toenails any more. So my grandfather does it for her all the time, even when his hands got arthritis, too. That's love.

- When someone loves you, the way she says your name is different. You know that your name is safe in her mouth.

- Life is "A." Love is the whole alphabet.

- Love is when a girl puts on perfume and a boy puts on shaving cologne and they go out and smell each other.

- Love is when you go out to eat and give somebody most of your French fries without making them give you any of theirs.

- Love is what makes you smile when you are tired.

- Love is when my mommy makes coffee for my daddy, and she takes a sip before giving it to him, to make sure the taste is OK.

- Love is when you kiss all the time. Then when you get tired of kissing, you still want to be together so you talk more. My mommy and daddy are like that. They look gross when they kiss, but they look happy and sometimes they dance in the kitchen while they're kissing.

- Love is what's in the room with you at Christmas if you stop opening presents for a minute and look around.

- Love is when Mommy gives Daddy the best piece of chicken.

- Love is when Mommy sees Daddy smelly and sweaty and still says he is handsomer than Robert Redford.

- If you want somebody to love you, then just be yourself. Some people try to act like somebody else, somebody the boy likes better. I think the boy isn't being very good if you feel this way and you should just find a nicer boy.

- Love is when your puppy licks your face even after you left him alone all day.

- When you're born and see your mommy the first time. That is love.

- Love goes on even when you stop breathing and you pick up where you left off when you reach heaven.

- You have to fall in love before you get married. Then when you are married, you just sit around and read books together.

- When you love somebody, your eyelashes go up and down and little stars come out of you.

- Love makes you sweat a lot.

- You can break love, but it won't die.

And one could do worse than to admire the quotations of seventeenth century poet and essayist Joseph Addison on the same subject:

- Admiration is a very short-lived passion that immediately decays upon growing familiar with its object, unless it be still fed with fresh discoveries, and kept alive by a new perpetual succession of miracles rising up to its view.

- Beauty soon grows familiar to the lover, fades in his eye, and palls upon the sense.

- A [hu]man must be both stupid and uncharitable who believes there is no virtue or truth but on his own side.

- The ideal [hu]man bears the accidents of life with dignity, and grace, the best of circumstances.

- I will indulge my sorrows, and give way to all the pangs and fury of despair. My death and life, my bane and antidote, are both before me.

- If [humans] would consider not so much where they differ, as wherein they agree, there would be far less of uncharitableness and angry feeling in the world.

- Through what variety of untried being, through what new scenes and changes must we pass! If you wish success in life, make perseverance your bosom friend, experience your wise counselor, caution your elder brother and hope your guardian genius.

- Three grand essentials to happiness in this life are something to do, something to love, and something to hope for.

- A [hu]man's first care should be to avoid the reproaches of his [or her] own heart.

- It is only imperfection that complains of what is imperfect. The more perfect we are, the more gentle and quiet we become towards the defects of others.

- Mysterious love, uncertain treasure, hast thou more of pain or pleasure? Endless torments dwell above thee: Yet who would live, and live without thee?

- But silence never shows itself to so great an advantage, as when it is made the reply to calumny and defamation.

* * *

On our honeymoon journey, Phil and I discovered the great taste of tempeh, an Indonesian fermented soy cake high in protein and isoflavones, which are known to strengthen bones, ease menopause symptoms, and reduce the risk of coronary heart disease and some cancers. We are both ambivalent toward tofu and were therefore pleasantly surprised by how much we liked the chewy, nutty flavor of these hearty patties, which can be cooked whole or cut into cubes and then crumbled to use in recipes as a meat substitute. Molds, mildews, and fungi stir up allergy symptoms in me, but I seem to be paradoxically tolerant of Rhizopus mold, the agent responsible for tempeh's fermentation process. It's important to remember to buy only the organic varieties that do not use genetically modified soybeans.

Being a vegetarian was no reason to give up the barbecue grill, especially now that we'd discovered tempeh, which, with a little barbecue sauce, a slice of cheddar, tomato, and lettuce makes a great "burger." Thankfully, Phil is adept at firing up the grill and experimenting with its effects on various recipes. Grilling fresh vegetables is not a new idea, but basting them in this tasty grilling sauce is. Phil thought the dish deserved an exotic name, so we chose "polou," the Iranian word for "rice dish" and served it alongside our tempeh "burgers."

Grilled Vegetable Polou

2-1/2 cups vegetable broth
1 cup uncooked brown basmati rice
1/2 teaspoon ground ginger
1 Walla Walla Sweet onion
1 green pepper
1 small eggplant
2 ripe tomatoes
2 tablespoons olive oil
1 tablespoon sunflower oil
1 tablespoon Trader Joe's Organic Red Wine and Olive Oil
    Vinaigrette
Pinch Tony Chachere's Original Creole Seasoning
Pinch garlic granules

Bring vegetable broth to a boil in a medium saucepan and add rice and ginger. Bring to a boil again, cover, and reduce heat to lowest setting. Simmer 50 minutes. Remove from heat and allow to sit undisturbed for 30 minutes. Meanwhile, cube and skewer vegetables. Mix remaining ingredients and brush on kebobs. Grill until edges of vegetables are brown, turning as needed. Remove from skewer and arrange on a bed of rice. Drizzle with remaining basting sauce. Makes two very generous portions.

*   *   *

And then there were the garlic scapes. Green as pastures, curly as sweet pea tendrils, but nothing compares to their strange flavorland, which is some place between horseradish and chives. Most places, they come into season in June, but in our region, July is the month. I would tell you more, but after the fashion of a good teacher, I want you to look them up. All but disguised in this flavorful summer soup, they are a sure cure for high blood pressure, unrequited desire, the hyperbole that is newlywed love, and sunburns. By the time we finished eating all this, we were full as ticks, but the world seemed unequivocally right.

Great (E)Scape Vichyssoise

3 tablespoons butter
3 tablespoons flour
3 cups vegetable broth
1 medium red potato, peeled and chopped
2 thick bunches scapes, finely chopped
Salt to taste
Paprika

Make a roux of butter and flour over low heat. Stir in broth a few tablespoons at a time to avoid lumps. Add potato and scapes, leaving a few scapes for garnish. Cook over low heat until potatoes are very, very soft, about 45 minutes, adding small amounts of additional broth as needed to keep mixture thinned. Allow to cool. Puree in blender. Salt to taste. Garnish with finely chopped raw scapes and a dash of paprika, and serve cold with grilled cheese triangles and watermelon wedges.

*   *   *

Laurel's Kitchen first crossed my path in the summer of 1980 while visiting friends in Corvallis, Oregon. I was quite pregnant with my oldest son, Sean, and was immediately drawn not only to its array of recipes—our hostess was serving Lasagne al Forno from its "Heartier Dishes" chapter—and depiction of the vegetarian lifestyle, but also its extensive nutrition information. Weeks later in Sisters, Oregon, while visiting in-laws, I found my own copy in a local bookstore. I never did know what my in-laws thought about me spending that weekend reading it from cover to cover. My interest in meditation and Zen Buddhism was also piqued during that original reading, and just thumbing through the book still has a soothing effect on me. As mentioned earlier, I have adapted Lasagne Al Forno so many times over the years that it has evolved into my own recipe. The sauce is the most flavorful and surprising I've ever tasted, especially compared to how flat store-bought tomato sauce of any kind is. I include it here again because we defrosted some on a hot July night to serve with rustic pasta from Italy we'd purchased on our "weddingmoon" at the Blue Heron French Cheese factory in Tillamook, Oregon. We served it cold and were surprised by how delicious it was that way. Any time I make this tomato sauce, I quadruple the batch and freeze it in two- to four-cup portions. I've canned many quarts of this versatile sauce, but freezing preserves the flavors and textures better. Many is the summer I have stood for days on end over a thirty-quart soup pot stirring garden-fresh acres of the stuff in preparation for its journey into quart jars and a hot-water bath in a large, blue-and-white speckled canning kettle. A cold packer, my mother used to call it. It is the herbs dried from fresh for the occasion—the fennel, the dried red chili seed, and the small bit of agave syrup—that catapults this traditional recipe into the realm of haute cuisine. Spike it with one half cup of hemp seed just prior to serving for a meatless protein boost.

Tomato Sauce

1/4 cup olive oil
2 medium red onions, chopped
4 cloves garlic, mashed
1 bell pepper, chopped
3 fresh bay leaves
2 tablespoons fresh oregano
1 tablespoon fresh thyme
1 tablespoon fresh basil
2 teaspoons fresh rosemary
2 teaspoons fennel seed
1/2 cup fresh parsley
2 tablespoons paprika

3 carrots, grated
6 cups chopped fresh tomatoes
2 6-ounce cans tomato paste
1 teaspoon ground pepper
1/4 teaspoon dried red chili seed
2 tablespoons agave syrup
Vegetable broth

Sauté onion, garlic, and pepper in olive oil until onion is transparent. Toss herbs in dry pan over medium heat until crumbly. Stir herbs and carrots into onion mix. Add tomatoes, paste, and seasonings. Thin with broth as needed. Cover and simmer for 20-30 minutes. For optimum flavor, rest in the refrigerator 24 hours before using.

* * *

And leave it to Phil to take that leftover pasta and tomato sauce, add artichoke hearts, a can of white beans, and Parmesan cheese and end up with a main course fit for company. It's not all that often I return for seconds, but that night I certainly did. If I had to put a name on it, I'd call it, "Tuscan White Bean Casserole." Yum.

* * *

LATE SUMMER DOWNPOUR

The rain picks at me like petals pulled adrift, easy
pinks, reds, and bright, sunbright, full of surprise, stark
wet and glistening even in moonlight, doubling
dew, and overnight settling of temperatures.
The sky quivers, shot full of lightning, then the quake,
black thunder, Rip Van Winkle sleeping through his
life's cartoon bowling alley, all those trolls with monstrous
biceps hurling sound enough to echo in my sleep, now
that I've soft-toed in my sleeping gown back up to bed,
having seen what the commotion was all about.

HWY. 195 BEFORE HARVEST

Somewhere in this lion's mane of wheat
is the birth of it, a kernel begetting
its own future, now thinking, who thought
to place me in such fertile ground? Who
empties the silos where I will eventually
end? Water is my closest neighbor but
no friend this late, this close to my great
transition. Such are the voices of growing
fields should any of us stop to listen passing by
on these wheat-free paved ways, hot oil
and gravel filling the ruts our roaring
wheels took all year to rout.

*   *   *

I think of fruit salad as a kind of free verse poem. With its entwined flavors—some sweet, some pungent—and textures—some staccato, some adagio—merging in unpredictable rhythms and deepened by the divine energies inherent in the reproductive imagery of fruit; it certainly inspires the creative. We all have grandmothers who laced their fruit salads with bits of marshmallow. Some folks like it spiked with a little rum. My Grandma Hazel jazzed hers with 7UP, an inspiration I've mimicked in the recipe below by making a sauce of sparkling mineral water, agave syrup, and lime, lemon, and pineapple juices. Huckleberries were yet to reach their peak season in our mountains, thanks to late snow and endless torrents of low temperatures and spring rain, so I had to rely on the previous year's frozen stores, and the last of the few we'd purchased from a local fruit vendor. I tried substituting blueberries, but it really was not the same. The chocolate mint we grew and dried ourselves.

We discovered chocolate mint in 2010 and keep two pots of it near the pond, since mint loves moisture, and it flourished in the spray coming off the waterfall—still flourishes, by the way, returning voluntarily in the same pot for three seasons now. Chocolate mint tastes and smells just as it sounds, with dark brown stalks and thick, chocolate-hued green leaves. It loves a little morning sun balanced by a lot of shade. The down-home name for the recipe is inspired by a regional dish made with pudding, JELL-O, and vanilla wafers known as "The Next Best Thing to Hugging Robert Redford." I very oddly ran across the dish at a friend's house in Oregon in 1998. It was the high priest of the Thanksgiving dessert table, and everyone was frantic to get through the turkey part to get their share. I took a dish of it just to get a good look since I coincidentally had just written a short story titled, "Hugging Robert Redford." It still seems weird to have had those three words repeated at me as the hostess, smiling and in slow motion, of course, handed me that sweet-smelling mishmash. The story was published several times, first in a literary journal called *Talking River Review* and then later in my short story collection, *Summer of Government Cheese.*

Next Stop Nirvana

1 cup huckleberries
2 bananas, sliced
1 nectarine, chopped
1 peach, chopped
1 12-ounce can pineapple chunks
1 cup walnut halves, coarsely chopped
2 tablespoons pineapple juice
2 teaspoons lemon juice
2 teaspoons lime juice
1 teaspoon agave syrup
1/2 cup San Pellegrino Sparkling Mineral Water
1/4 cup candied ginger, finely chopped
2 tablespoons chocolate mint leaves, crushed
1 ounce dark chocolate, grated
Honey

Mix fruits and walnuts in medium-sized bowl. Mix juices, agave syrup, and water, pour over fruit and toss lightly with ginger and mint leaves. Separate into serving bowls, top with grated chocolate, and drizzle lightly with honey. Garnish with dark chocolate wafer cookies and serve immediately, else the sauce loses its fizz. Makes 4 good-sized helpings, or, 8-12 if split up over scoops of sherbet.

*   *   *

"Quite skeptical" aptly describes my response to the young woman at the Moscow Food Co-op bulk food bins who, upon revealing that she and her husband had recently become vegetarians, described a recipe she had tried called Cottage Cheese Burgers. When she mentioned the word husband, I had to extinguish an urge to tell her I was newly wed after twenty years of being single and that it occasionally made me want to kill something—primarily my new husband. I wanted to tell her how I felt—or imagined I felt—a new expectation from him that I was to have dinner ready when he got home from work, about how quickly I started accusing him of having forgotten that I am a writer, not a wife, not a housekeeper. About how little time had passed before we'd torn off our wedding rings, stashed them in a drawer, and I'd moved downstairs into the guest bedroom. About how, one week when he had to be gone for training, I removed every reminder of him, including his family pictures, and stashed them in a drawer. A rage was the word I would use.

Instead, I told her that in all my years of reading organic and vegetarian food cookbooks and magazines, Cottage Cheese Burgers had never presented themselves. She insisted I Google them, which I did (that virtual verb most of us grew up knowing only as a theoretical number) and found a crazy-large array of related recipes, although not quite a google of them. They might be an acquired taste for some, but we dressed them up in our own way and found them flavorful and oddly satisfying as a burger substitute, a thing for which we obviously were homesick.

Oatmeal/Cottage Cheese Burgers

    1 cup cottage cheese
    2 cups oats
    1 medium-sized red potato, boiled
    2 eggs, slightly beaten
    1 medium onion
    1 cup walnuts, ground
    Unbleached flour
    Fresh ground black pepper
    Tony Chachere's Original Creole Seasoning

Place all ingredients except flour and seasonings in food processor and combine. Scoop into a medium-sized bowl. Add unbleached flour by hand as necessary to thicken into a moldable consistency. Allow to rest in the refrigerator 30 minutes. Form into patties. Season lightly on each side. Fry or grill. Serve on buns with your favorite condiments, cheese, lettuce, and tomatoes.

* * *

The birth of my son Sean in August, 1980, sparked for me an interest in nutrition and organic food that was fueled by monthly issues of *Mother Earth News* and trips to the library to check out books on everything from composting to drying and preserving food. During those first years of his life, he ate almost nothing that I did not grow, pick, purchase in bulk and/or preserve. No white sugar. No white flour. Baby food ground by hand, frozen in little cubes, and stored in cottage cheese containers labeled with masking tape. I still remember being upset when, at age two, someone gave him COOL WHIP. His father, a veteran hunter, brought home every manner of game from birds to elk and deer to wild-caught fish. Somewhere during my pregnancy, I read about the relationship between brain and neuro-system development and a pregnant woman's consumption of fish. Since we almost always had a supply of steelhead fillets in the freezer, I assumed Sean's level of intelligence came as a direct result of his father's fishing habit. I like to think early good nutrition created in him a sense of stability, a penchant for healthy habits, and an awareness of the connection between well-being and food. He still insists the deprivation merely created in him a candy addiction. Ah, well. I was at least forty before I made a trip to see my parents to tell them I had finally figured out I needed to give credit where credit was due.

In August 2010, I was more concerned with strawberries ripening quite late thanks, again, to the long spring and cool summer, or it might have been the result of growing them in ceramic pots on the deck sequestered by wire mesh to keep the squirrels off. Either way, that year's strawberries were just not as tasty as we had expected, given their shock-red color and the Alpine variety's reputation for sweetness. Nor were they abundant. We finally removed the wire covers and added strawberries to the list of things we grow and never get to consume because of the squirrels: chestnuts, apples, Concord grapes, crabapples, mulberries, and walnuts, not to mention the holly berries that make them drunk at Christmas, the Oregon grape, and whatever the tiny green berries are hanging from the shrubs on the south side of the deck, the even tinier seeds of which they crack open, leaving the scattered shells for us to sweep. The entertainment value of squirrels as they chase around the yard courting and mating, playing games, rearing and training their young, nibbling on the bread crumbs and stale crackers we leave for them, of course, being worth the sacrifice.

I love the final days of summer when there is every reason to sit around watching the unmoving leaves, avoiding doing all the things we need to be doing. Sun. Heat. No wind. All of a sudden it is okay to drop everything and head for the mountains. All of a sudden it is okay not to care whether the lawn needs mowing. All of a sudden it is okay to sit inside the kitchen nook windows watching a squirrel, one of the first we'd seen in the yard since before the wedding, and apparently new to the neighborhood, going insane over the pond, the waterfall, the bounty of fruit and nuts and sycamore balls. All of a sudden it is okay to while away the hours of a day doing absolutely only whatever a soul is inclined to do. If you do make yourself get up and mow the lawn, you have the perfect excuse for a cold treat: the candy-red of watermelon's sweetmeat. Eaten straight from jewel-green and cream rinds, it is also a color feast. But for some reason that wasn't enough on this particular day, and so Phil and I, feeling extraordinarily decadent and deserving, headed to Baskin-Robbins, only to discover watermelon sherbet laced with dark chocolate "seeds," an instantaneous addiction I ended up fighting for a month, sneaking off to the BR every few days to indulge myself. I don't know why it is that near the end of August, right before time for the new fall semester starts, I don't want to eat anything but popsicles and ice cream, but it is true.

By Labor Day, and nearly the end of camping season, sticking to a vegetarian diet was much less intimidating, and we were adjusting to our new situation. All cozied into a spot on Chesnimus Creek in the Wallowa-Whitman National Forest, marveling briefly over the obnoxious power a piece of paper printed with the words "Marriage Certificate" had to trigger ingrained social expectations—even when they are against personal convictions—we drizzled olive oil, hemp seed, and butter over a medley of red potatoes and vegetables, sealed it in foil, and threw it on the fire for a satisfying accompaniment to cottage cheese and a can of organic pineapple.

The weekend prior, at the same magical spot, graced that time with visits from a snowshoe hare in his summer coat and several hummingbirds attracted to the red labels on all our various pieces of Coleman gear, Phil made stir-fry magic with several cups of white basmati we'd cooked and packed ahead, farmer's market veggies, and a quarter cup or so of hemp seed. We found ourselves having to be a bit more creative about preparations than we ordinarily would. Perhaps it was this intensified prep work that caused us to forget our new eighteen-inch deep airbed and the little camp percolator we fell so in love with on our Lochsa River trip. We both felt a bit proud of the fact that, at fifty-two and fifty-three, we were able to sleep two nights in a row virtually on the ground, padded only by half an inch of closed-cell foam and a couple of wool blankets. Not to mention the great cowboy coffee we made, simply by boiling ground coffee and running it through a strainer lined with paper towels. Necessity being the mother of all invention.

*　*　*

Chop wood; carry water, the Buddha said. I've always taken that to mean, "Look for the spiritual in the mundane." I found myself feeling centered and peaceful, preparing for our final camping trip the following weekend while making cannelloni—including the noodles—from scratch. The recipe was quite simple: two cups unbleached organic flour mixed with one half teaspoon salt, two unbeaten eggs, one half cup water. And unorthodox. I placed the flour in a steep mound right on the kitchen counter's surface, made a well, put the eggs in the well, and started working them into the flour with my fingers, adding the water a bit at a time. The challenge was in keeping the eggs off the counter. Once I had a dough, I kneaded it for five minutes or so, then let it rest for ten before dividing it in half, powdering the counter with more flour, and rolling the dough out to one sixteenth of an inch thick. Of course, some people use a pasta machine, but the reward for all that finger work was deciding on dough shapes, cutting the dough uniformly, in this case four-by-six-inch squares for stuffing with cheeses and rolling into tubes. I could have just as easily cut it into squares for ravioli or long rectangles for lasagna. I also could have cut it into strips or various other noodle shapes, which later could have been dried. The difference in flavor and texture when compared to packaged pasta was, of course, mind-boggling, and as a consequence I've repeated the process several times since.

Why did we all switch to factory-prepared foods? If we'd only start realizing, as a culture, what we are missing by not placing at the center of our existences the growing and preparing of food. I'm convinced all our mental and physical health issues would simply float away. Doctors would have to go back to playing golf on Wednesdays and giving out lollipops to attract customers. I say this because, as a bonus, the mixing, kneading, and rolling was somewhat aerobic, evidenced by the generous sweat I worked up. Enough to counter the fat calories from all that cheese in the final product, which we relished out there under that section of primitive, blue, private sky.

* * *

Every year from 1991 to 2008, on the first day of September, my long-time friend Bob and I would either call or email each other to say, "It's September." A ritual which started simply because, not too long after meeting in July 1991, at Oregon's now defunct Wallowa Lake Jazz Festival, we both admitted to feeling a sigh of relief once September arrived. I am a September baby, born the twenty-ninth; Bob was a mid-autumn baby, born November 3rd. We shared a love for autumn, for the changing colors and dropping of leaves, for the world growing quiet and dim and restful. He was one of those friends who always seemed to know when I was suffering, his phone calls to assess my well-being coming alongside my brother Jacob's, who regularly successfully senses when I need a shoulder on which to lean.

Bob died on August 4, 2009, of cancer, after an eighteen-month fight in which everyone who knew him sought to keep him alive with potions and incantations. His caregiver said it was like an endless parade of shamans coming through the front door, each with his or her sure cure: vitamins and nutritional supplements; exotic fungi. Plus our donation of hemp seed oil and powder. Bob himself sought out therapies from a Portland-based clinic specializing in flower essences as a cancer treatment. In the end, it was words that killed him, a nay-saying physician who said, "You are a fool. You need to be getting your affairs in order." After more than a year of keeping himself alive by the power of faith and will and the love of his friends, within a week of that sentence being uttered, Bob was dead.

That Bob should die of cancer stunned all of us who knew him. He had done everything right, in fact could have been the proverbial poster child for "doing it right." He had kept himself physically very fit, practiced meditation and yoga, used his bike as his primary source of transportation, was active in trying to preserve wildlands, and had a tremendous respect for the natural world and all its creatures. He ate mostly organic foods, very little meat—virtually none of it red—and was well known for eschewing anything processed. He even refused to eat movie theater popcorn, threatening on more than one occasion to take a bag of kale to the movies—or so the legend goes.

Several weeks after he had died—it was not quite September 1, I remember, but almost—Phil and I (Phil mostly) finally had gotten around to opening a box of solar-powered yard lights from Costco we'd purchased during the summer, glass bulbs that were supposed to shift from red to blue to green encased in bronze crescent moons and suns. It was after dark when Phil opened those boxes, which were sealed at the factory and shrink-wrapped in plastic. We sat on our deck talking about Bob's wake, from which we had just returned, wondering aloud whether we would indeed have a sign that he was trying to reach out to us from beyond. A deal I have jokingly made over the years with several friends—if you go first, and there is any way to communicate with me, you damned well better get through to me and let me know you are okay. At that moment, all four yard lights suddenly burst into bright-bright color, two blue and two red, and stayed that way as if trying to force themselves into our open-mouthed, awe-stricken awareness. How on earth? Well, obviously not of this earth as we later concluded, since never again have they glowed that brightly or failed to change colors. In fact, to this day we get almost no glow from those things at all on overcast days, and they come on gradually, and one at a time, never all at once. To our minds, there was absolutely only one way for solar batteries more than a year inside a cardboard box (if the manufacturing and shipping date could be believed) to launch themselves into such a raucous display: it was simply Bob, making his ethereal rounds, saying his goodbyes, perhaps even letting us know just how much fun it is to be on the other side. I mention Bob because I eventually turned to flower essences to deal with some of the emotional stress I was feeling and to minimize what I was starting to suspect might be some sort of mild post-traumatic stress. The school year was coming on again, and despite the fact that we were nine months into our first year as vegetarians, stress and its ability to lower blood sugar was once again taking us by surprise. One day later in September, Phil called to say somewhat frantically that he was headed into town from his office, a fifteen-mile distance, to Taco Time for a Vegetarian Burrito. He wanted to know if I would join him.

"I can't take it," he said, "I have to eat."

It was nearing the end of the fiscal year, his busiest and most difficult time, and he was forced to work a considerable amount of overtime, suffering sleep interruptions at night, presumably from stress. I was feeling similarly ravenous and unable to focus, having at the end of August begun the new semester of classes at my university teaching job. My stomach had been against my backbone all day, and our daily quart of hemp shake just wasn't cutting it.

We have one of the best Taco Times in the world, owned by the father of a friend of ours who has a chain of local places such as The Main Street Grill, Zany Graze, and Tomato Brothers, and who some years ago gutted the place and had it restored to mimic a Mexican Hacienda. We love the decor and trust the food's quality because it is made with regional and fresh ingredients. Not a bad lunch for two people for less than ten dollars: two vegetarian burritos and a medium order of those infamous Mexi-Fries, which I used to cook regularly when my sons were young and which you can still find frozen in a plastic bag in just about any grocery store, under the name "Tater Tots." They are, unequivocally, the ultimate comfort food.

Phil mused over lunch that perhaps it was going to be a hard winter, since for days neither of us had wanted to do anything but eat. I kept trying to convince him it was an issue of stress for him and increased activity for me, since classes were back in session, and I was back to hiking almost two miles a day just to get to my office and back from where I had to park my car. If the layer of fat the squirrels were developing was any indication, however, he was going to end up right. The pair chasing each other across the yard when I got back home were the size of rodeo steers, and when Phil got home from work that night, I told him so.

*　*　*

Ah, the luxury of coming home on a cool, October evening to a pot of navy beans cooked earlier in the week and a stack of garden-fresh tomatoes from one of the final Saturday farmer's markets of the season. The requisite accompaniment? A pan of cornbread, of course. This is the recipe I watched both my grandmothers make, neither of them ever touching a measuring cup or spoon. I've added my own touches, of course: the yogurt and sunflower oil are meant to take the place of lard; chilis and cumin add texture and a bit of bite; the agave syrup heightens the chili flavor. Heartwarming enough for the last days of October ushering in a thirty-degree-temperature drop.

Grandma's Panbread

6 handfuls cornmeal
6 handfuls flour
3 tilts of the sunflower oil bottle
2 large dollops plain yogurt
1 6-ounce can chopped Hatch green chilies
1 pinch salt
2 pinches baking powder
1 pinch baking soda
1 pinch ground cumin
1 squirt agave syrup
Milk, enough to make a thick batter
2 egg whites

Preheat oven to 325 degrees. Mix all ingredients except
egg whites just until lumps dissolve. Do not over-stir
and do not beat. Whisk egg whites to foam. Fold gently
into batter. Pour mixture into buttered cast iron skillet.
Bake until toothpick comes out clean and bread pulls
from the side of the pan, 45-60 minutes. Allow to cool to
room temperature. Serve with soft butter and honey.

* * *

I'm here today to talk about a good-ol'-boy phenomenon known
as beer-can chicken. It may seem odd to tout a means for preparing
meat in a space meant for exploring vegetarianism, but I would be
remiss in not reminding my audience that healthy meat is available,
if you are willing to spend the time, effort, and money required to
seek it out. Our farmer's market always has locally raised animal
carcasses for sale—carcasses of naturally hypertrophied muscle,
naturally hypertrophied because the animal actually had to walk from
spot to spot to feed him- or herself. This process is known as free
grazing or, in organic-ese, "range-fed." In chickens, this process is
referred to as "free-range," which is not the same as "cage-free." Cage-
free birds may still be cramped into disastrous living situations which
render them too heavy to even support their own weight and in which
several of them succumb daily simply because they drop to the ground
and are suffocated by the bodies of their coop-mates. They are not happy
chickens. Happy chickens run around farmyards, flirting with roosters.

In preparation for an autumn celebration weekend with my son Sean,
his wondrous wife Susannah, and my two heart-melting granddaughters,
Phil and I purchased and froze a fresh-off-the-feet bird from our local
Saturday farmer's market, of the free-range, vegetarian-fed, organic
variety. We were all headed into the mountains to McCall, Idaho, to
spend a few days in a rented cabin. Sean and Susannah would cook a
vegetarian meal; we would cook a meat-based meal with a vegetarian
side dish. Fortune being the bold beast that it is, they had given us for
Christmas the previous year a device for making "beer-can chicken"—
sold at sporting goods stores and consisting of a piece of metal mesh
supporting a ring several inches high and just the right diameter to

hold a twelve-ounce beer can (and the cheaper the beer the better, or so we've been told)—just in time for us to decide to turn vegetarian. One of the last meat dishes we ate, in fact, was beer-can chicken, although snoots that we are, we used an empty soda can that we'd filled with a dark, rich porter. Simply massage the chicken with butter and sprinkle it with garlic powder and a bit of Tony Chachere's Original Creole Seasoning, impale the chicken on the beer can, set the contraption on the charcoal grill, drop the lid in place, and wait. The result, after about an hour of cooking is tender, juicy chicken.

Missing a grill, we improvised at the cabin with an inverted soup pot, then inserted the first can of Budweiser I have purchased in two decades into the device, perched Mr. Real Chicken—looking for all the world like a man in a tuxedo—on his final perch, and placed the works on a broiling pan in the oven on the lowest rack at 300 degrees. It took about an hour. The smell was tantalizing, I have to admit. Sean and Susannah not only loved it but were happy to take the leftovers home, and Phil was having a bit of a time not diving in. Unfortunately, and I speak from experience, since this is my second go at the vegetarian lifestyle, a person who hasn't eaten meat in a while can suffer painful, gouty joints, stomach aches, intestinal cramps, and well, use your imagination from there. . Papaya enzyme is a good digestive aid to counter these symptoms, but some people actually have no trouble at all.

She'd been considering it for some time, but after that meal and some encouragement and instruction, Susannah decided to make the switch to using organic foods, which is salve for my worried grandmother heart and a decision that has been in the making for a while. I still tremble at the thought of that permanently pink Walmart ground beef. Just one more frightening thing about the times in which we live. If ever an evil dictator wanted to control masses of humans, feeding them non-food, giving them swirly-gigs to keep them so mesmerized they don't want to move off the couch, making them believe that "Googling" is learning, then making it so expensive to fix their impaired bodies once they start breaking down that only the very affluent can afford to do so and only the poor die off would be one way to do it.

While Sean and Susannah were out with the girls and I was searching for words to describe in a poem our weekend and the mountains of Idaho in autumn in general, Phil whipped up a nice little rice and vegetable dish to use up the mountains of fresh, organic produce we had purchased at the Farmer's Market in McCall that Saturday. A balance of heat and intense basil paired with slices of Australian red pepper cheese on the side and cubed watermelon after, this simple meal was as satisfying as it was delectable and easy.

My list of descriptors for my poem? Stonewashed sky; woodsmoke; sweater-cool; raincoat mornings; hot cocoa; tomato-lined windows; apricot pie; football; steaming breath; shock-orange leaves, damp and molting; weed stubble; deepening nights; mothballed quilts.

Hot Tomato-Basil Casserole

2 cups water
1 cup uncooked brown basmati rice
2 pounds fresh tomatoes, chopped
5 cloves garlic, minced
1/2 cup fresh basil, chopped
1 Walla Walla Sweet onion, chopped
1 yellow squash, chopped
1/8 teaspoon fresh ground pepper
1/8 teaspoon Tony Chachere's Original Creole Seasoning
Saltines

Preheat oven to 350. Heat water to boiling. Add rice. Cover and cook on very low heat for 45 minutes. Meanwhile, stew tomatoes, garlic, basil, and onion, adding water as necessary to maintain a medium sauce. Simmer covered on very low heat for 20 minutes. Add squash. Season to taste. Layer rice and tomato mixture alternately with crumbled saltines at least twice in baking dish. Bake for 20 minutes. Allow to rest 10 minutes and serve.

* * *

I would prefer not to hike right on top of fresh, dark-purple-from-all-those-autumn-berries bear scat or giant bear footprints. But if it's likely that I'll have to run for my life, it's nice to know I'm fully fueled by Maui Mix, my new favorite kind of gorp. It's not our idea, but our recipe. The original version on which Maui Mix is based is called Tropical Mix. We bought it at the quick stop in Anatone, Washington, on the way to Field's Spring for a two-mile hike that was to turn into nearly a three-hour one because we didn't have a map and the trail crisscrossed so many times that if we did have a map it would be about as readable as tea leaves. And then there was the possibility of that bear, of course, which kept us singing "In-A-Gadda-Da-Vida"—loudly and badly enough to run off just about anything—all the way back down the mountain and until we were safely inside the Subaru.

Maui Mix

2 cups dried pineapple pieces, chopped
2 cups banana chips
2 cups organic toffee peanuts
2 cups organic sesame wheat sticks
2 cups whole, raw almonds

Roast almonds on a baking sheet at 225 degrees for 2 hours. Cool then chop. Mix all ingredients. Store in sealed container.

* * *

Stress did finally spawn disease, but not in me. Even a vegetarian diet was not enough to keep Phil off the examining table late in November—a paralytic ileus, the sequelae of a diverticulitis attack. A word of warning: chronic discomfort in the lower left side of the abdomen almost always means a diverticulum has developed, an out pocketing of the intestinal wall designed just right to catch bits of food, much as happens with the appendix. Pain sufficient to awaken a person at night or when lying on the left side means the thing is inflamed and will require a course of antibiotics to heal it. If it bursts, the result is a hospital stay and very likely surgery, and in the worst cases, death. Diverticulitis—or any pelvic inflammation—can cause portions of the bowel to shut down, usually the ileus, which is the lower portion of the small intestine just above where it connects to the colon. Symptoms include foul breath or a bad taste in the mouth; abnormal, frequent, loud belching; narrowed stool (pencil- to finger-sized); and gurgling in the intestines. The narrowed stools are a good and bad sign. They mean the bowel is only partially blocked, but they also mean the bowel *is* partially blocked. A fully blocked bowel is an emergency and can result in death within hours. Paralytic ileus can also be caused by blood clots, fat embolism, abdominal scar tissue, and cancer. Treatment for all and any of the above ranges from ten days of two or more high-powered broad-spectrum antibiotics to surgery resulting in temporary or permanent colostomy. Think of the intestinal system as an auto's intake, combustion, and exhaust system. Interfere at any stage of the process and see what happens when you try to operate your vehicle. The human body is exactly the same, and the thing that keeps it in shape is to keep it moving, literally and figuratively—exercise and a high-fiber diet are your gut's best friends. Our hero Phil would do well to incorporate a daily walk into his life plan. Happily, his CT scan showed no signs of abdominal cancer, but that high-fibered hemp protein had to be put on the sidelines in favor of first a liquid diet, then a soft one. Cream soups, cottage cheese, white bread, and applesauce.

And what are the primary metaphysical causes of a blocked bowel?

Anger, guilt, and fear. And because it's on the left side—holding oneself back.

Because I was worried that nuts might also be a culprit, since in the old days we were trained that nuts and seeds had to be excluded from the diets of people with diverticulosis, I started turning all the nuts we were using to offset low blood sugars into nut butters. All of a sudden we had an exciting new repertoire of snack possibilities. I instantly became stuck on sunflower butter. The vaguely tawny, thin spread is perfect for dipping a celery stick or oat cracker. And if I applaud Monterey Jack cheese and sunflower butter grilled on potato sourdough, I'll also have to applaud Bloodroot Stew, which is the only logical accompaniment, and as elegant as only autumn dishes on cool, overcast, late November evenings can be.

Bloodroot Stew with Grilled Sunflower Sandwiches

Stew:

3 pounds baby beets, peeled and halved
1 large Walla Walla Sweet onion, very coarsely chopped
6 cloves elephant garlic, muddled
2 pounds freshly picked young carrots, sliced
2 pounds baby red potatoes, halved
Sandwiches:
4 slices fresh, artisan potato sourdough bread
4 tablespoons butter
2 full slices Monterey Jack cheese
2 tablespoons sunflower butter

Blanch first 5 ingredients in 1 quart water for 10 minutes. Cover and simmer until beets are soft. Allow to rest 15 minutes.

While stew is resting, melt 2 tablespoons butter on griddle. For each sandwich: take two slices of bread and spread 1-1/2 tablespoons butter on one side of each slice. Place non-buttered side down onto melted butter on griddle. When the griddle sides are browned, flip the slices. Spread 1 tablespoon sunflower butter on the browned side of one slice; place cheese slices on the browned side of the other slice. Put cheese side and sunflower butter side of sandwich together. Continue grilling sandwich on both sides, flipping regularly, until both are evenly brown. Serves 4 half-sandwiches and 4 plentiful bowls of stew.

* * *

And so Phil found himself facing the long alleyway between himself and optimum health. Diagnosed with full-blown diabetes, low B-12 levels (a risk with vegetarian diets), extremely low Vitamin D (five years of living in the northwest), clinical depression, and high blood pressure, the doctors told him diverticulitis was only part of his worries: he was also at severe risk for early heart attack or stroke. I had not wanted to mention to him the word depression, but our fighting had increased as the days grew shorter, and when he told me twice in one week that he wished he weren't even alive, I stepped up to the plate and dragged him to a see a doctor—as much as I did not want to turn him over to allopathic cures. Funny, I could trust my health to downhome therapies, but not his. Which translated to, of course, a mountain of pharmaceuticals. You know life has changed when you find yourself heading to the drugstore for a monthly pill organizer. We balked at the doctor's insisting on a flu shot—both of us doubting the wisdom in messing with the body's immune system. But since we were buying into part of the medical-industrial complex's recommendations, we decided to buy into all of it, and Phil did indeed roll up his sleeve for the injection. People with diabetes do tend to get more infections. I had been nursing my father long distance for years for all these same issues. I guess you could say I was well rehearsed; still, I couldn't help but be troubled. A dream right before I met Phil featured a guy with a colostomy who was trying to get into my pants. Sick, right? A guy with shit-in-a-bag hanging from his belly trying to seduce me on a ratty mattress in an old warehouse. That dream was all I could think about. I do not like nursing sick people. Selfish, selfish, I know. But I was just so freaking exhausted from it all. And now this.

And poor Phil. In the middle of one big self-pity party, himself, and who could blame him? Once again our nights became one sobbing mutual rant after another sobbing mutual rant: mythic, apocalyptic, emotional blowouts. And why? For what? I think for me, I hated that stupid piece of paper and its implied ownership. For both of us, I think we were figuratively arguing with our ex-spouses, picking up where we left off with unfinished business, blaming each other for everything that had ever gone wrong in our lives. Those evenings meant going through my days feeling wrung out as on old dishrag. Still struggling with the lung infection all those months later, angry at myself, really, for having fallen into a marriage again when I had so enjoyed my freedom. (But I was done with it! I wanted this!) Discontent swelled like huge beestings inside my heart and lungs. (And yes, I know, mixed metaphors. But the occasion calls for it.) Which played itself out in me as diarrhea — cathartic and frequent enough to be called a mantra.

* * *

Then. Finally. Finally. One night it came.

How on earth the body can keep producing so much saltwater over so much time, I don't know. The amount of fluid and hours spent rehashing the past year's frustrations were enough to gestate, birth, and age another entire human. And what we were both raging against was our own selves. Afraid of our own damned failures. Of this new frontier hurting us in the same way, and for me — again.

And of course there is more I'm not telling.

But in the end, we came to this awareness: it was true we were standing by each other only tangentially, but it was also true that we still each felt a teeny-tiny little ghost flame from what had once been for both of us our life's most intense connection with another human. I said to Phil point blank that I knew I would continue to offer at least a small measure of support as long as he kept his health as his first concern, but I was not going to live with a man who did not love himself enough to take care of himself. What I knew I felt for him was the uncommon bond of real friendship. Not the brand of friendship drinking buddies share or people who engage in common interests or activities. But the sort of friendship people who are interested in the well-being of each other share.

* * *

But then came Christmas dinner. We had all the kids in — Sean, Susannah, Malory, Leah, who was nearing a year old, Jacob, Kelsey, and Aaron, who was almost three months. Phil cooked his famous, succulent, prime rib rimed with rock salt. I made a gravy done the down-home way, with browned flour and butter to form what more sophisticated folks might call a dark roux, did my even more famous mashed potatoes: five pounds of potatoes to a half pound of butter and real, full-fat cream, not half and half, not milk.

The smell was so soul-grabbing even I had to try the gravy, but Phil swallowed a few papaya capsules bought in anticipation and ate the animal flesh. Symbolic, I thought, of the two of us and the silly gulf that had existed between us for months, to which we were clearly both simply clinging, the way a possum baby clings to its mother. But he might as well have had sex with somebody else on the table right in front of me. I couldn't get the sight out of my mind of the fork laden with meat-dripping-juice entering his face. And that was to be just the beginning.

Phil once again started buying and cooking animal flesh. Our food bill skyrocketed. It might have been an over-reaction, but I found I could no longer stand the feel of his touch, nor he mine, apparently. The wedding rings remained in their box. We talked about burning the marriage license. Our together time came down to watching television. Phil seethed with something I couldn't stand to be near. Aggression. Cynicism. I devolved into a steamy porridge of bitterness and self-loathing, staying late at work, leaving home to write and work in coffee shops. I thought of Jill's visits to assist people in Haiti, striving so courageously to survive a massive earthquake, and with scant resources and disease. I thought of Tesla, so intent on escaping from a situation in which he did not belong. In which he wasn't allowed the freedom to roam. Maybe the freedom to roam was the answer. After a lifetime of living through trials and tragedies, even toxic mold, and the mere act of exchanging wedding bands had done me in. And screw perseverance. Now we didn't even have food in common.

*   *   *

"One quarter of what you eat keeps you alive. The other three-quarters keeps your doctor alive."

—Ancient Egyptian Proverb

Thankfully for us and me and our relationship, once again, Phil's body stepped in. Animal flesh is murder on colons. In fact, look up diverticulitis and find testimony after testimony of people on high-protein-from-animal-flesh diets developing colon symptoms. Phil struggled with diverticulitis until one night we "Googled it" (that blasphemous phrase again, and I say blasphemous because surely the gods of research libraries must hate it for luring us out of the stacks the way it has) and found testimony after testimony about a miracle cure: aloe vera juice. And miracle is the apt word because half a cup of the faintly greenish tasting stuff was all it took to calm his throbbing colon. And daily doses have kept it calm. For nearly two years now. If secretions from aloe vera's puffy "leaves" can regenerate skin after a burn, surely it must do wonders for an inflamed gut.

During that same week, Phil picked up a film called *Forks Over Knives* about the work of two researchers, Dr. T. Colin Campbell and Dr. Caldwell B. Esselstyn, Jr., on the relationship between food and health. Some highlights from the film:

- We spend $2.2 trillion per year on health care in the U.S., which is five times what we spend on the military.

- We all suffer from chronic fatigue derived from nutrition deficits and mask it with coffee, sugar, and high-energy drinks.

- We spend $50 billion a year in the U.S. on coronary bypasses.

- In laboratory studies, animal protein has been shown to "turn on" cancer cells.

- During WWII, the Germans confiscated all cows and pigs in Norway and heart disease dropped by astonishing rates, then came back up after hostilities ended and animal proteins were reintroduced.

- The 1973 farm subsidy bill resulted in increased corn production and widespread use of high-density corn syrup.

- Stretch receptors in the stomach help to gauge how much we've eaten and density receptors measure caloric content or richness. Five hundred calories of plant food fills the stomach completely and satisfies density receptors sending the message to our stomachs that we've had enough to eat. Five hundred calories of processed food only fills the stomach halfway, which is not enough to satisfy density receptors. Five hundred calories of fat doesn't satisfy either.

- Human beings are motivated by three things: pleasure (food, sex), avoidance of pain, and energy conservation. Richer food excites motivational sensors because it gives the greatest amount of food with the least amount of effort. This helped our ancestors seek the most calorie-dense and ripe foods available, which worked to ensure our survival. Today's foods give us an excessive amount of pleasure when compared to those found in nature, which leads us to what is referred to as "the pleasure trap." The pleasure trap works like drugs because it hijacks the pleasure cycle. Rich and processed foods hyperconcentrate sugar and fat in such a way that what we are all struggling with is a low-grade addiction. This phenomenon preys on the less affluent who have little choice but to buy cheap food and who use food to fill emotional gaps left by poverty, such as low self-esteem.

- In China in the 1970s, Premier Zhou Enlai ordered the systematic interviewing of 880,000,000 people to research the mortality patterns of certain kinds of cancers. Six hundred fifty thousand researchers compiled information on 367 diet and nutritional variables which were published as a sort of "cancer atlas" in 1981. The results showed clear cancer hotspots that directly correlated to the consumption of animal protein. Dr. Campbell and physicians from China subsequently took urine and blood samples from 6,500 rural Chinese in sixty-five Chinese counties and discovered 94,000 correlations between diet and disease. The evidence was irrefutable: people who ate nearest to a one hundred percent plant-based diet had the least amount of cancer, diabetes, and heart disease. In fact, almost none. Thirty years later, what we know is that the wide-spread availability of American fast foods in China has brought with it the wide-spread incidence of the Western world's three main causes of death: diabetes, cancer, and heart disease.

- At the same time, Dr. Esselstyn began a study with twenty-four subjects, all of whom had significant heart disease, including two with failed bypass surgeries and five who'd been given death sentences. All were treated first with a vegetarian diet, which included dairy and eggs, and later with a one hundred percent plant-based diet. Of the eighteen who stayed with the study for the full five years, all had complete reversals of their heart disease, all were still living two decades—twenty years!—later, and all were still sexually active. (Erectile dysfunction is often the first sign of heart disease.) What we know about blood vessels is that the cells lining them (endothelial cells) normally produce nitrous oxide, which keeps blood flowing, keeps inflammation down, and inhibits the production of plaque. Plaque is made of cholesterol, which the body manufactures but we also consume in meat and dairy products. Plaque buildup is rough, and when blood cells hit it, they release clotting factor. Clotting factor is a good thing if you've skinned your knee. Throw some into a blood vessel narrowed by plaque, and you've got a heart attack or a stroke. The Western diet slaughters endothelial cells, but a plant-based diet restores them.

- Dr. Esselstyn removed dairy from his patients' diets when he realized that people who eat high levels of dairy products suffer high rates of hip fractures. It turns out that animal products create a condition in the body called metabolic acidosis. The body balances metabolic acidosis by hailing its most accessible acid buffer: calcium from the bones.

- The relationship between the use of low-fat dairy products and prostate cancer is as straightforward as the relationship between smoking tobacco and lung cancer. Put bluntly, prostate cancer skyrockets among men who use low-fat dairy products.

- Plant proteins failed to support cancers in animals in laboratory studies: in fact, nutrients from plants consistently decrease cancer growth.

*   *   *

Anybody can guess the rest. We bought a book called *Vegan Cooking for Dummies*, and I found an extraordinary website called "Oh She Glows" out of Canada created by a young woman who switched to the vegan lifestyle but refused to give up gourmet cooking. We now make her veggie burgers by the triple batch. We learned about substituting half a banana for the egg in bread, cookie, muffin, and pancake recipes and two tablespoons of ground flax seed soaked in a quarter-cup of warm water in everything else. We discovered that we actually liked Vegenaise better than traditional mayo and that a product called Earth Balance keeps us from missing butter. We use hazelnut milk instead of cow's milk. Tried almond-milk and soy cheeses and found them if not every bit as satisfying and functional in recipes as regular cheese, at least a palatable substitute. At this point we are using almost no processed foods, so we rarely buy those, unless we have a real hankering for mac 'n' cheese. We even recently began juicing.

What we found ourselves craving, oddly enough, was fish, so for most of 2012, we adhered to the Chinese tradition of ninety-five percent vegan—which is also the Haitian tradition, it turns out—reasoning that three or four ounces of wild-caught northern water fish every few weeks to bolster our omegas and protein intake might not hurt. I thought that compared to just about how often I might be able to catch a fish if I lived in the wilderness. And although I reduced the amount of organic half-and-half I take in my morning cup of organic-fair-trade-shade-grown-coffee to one tablespoon and substitute coconut milk for the rest, I am so far unwilling to give up that one tiny thing, and as long as I only have one or two smallish cups of coffee, I don't get ear infections. What I've discovered after removing dairy otherwise from my diet, is a sensitivity to gluten (I thought my propensity for naps was fatigue; turns out fatigue is sometimes the only symptom of sensitivity to gluten) so, as much as possible, we go for gluten-free.

Somewhere in there I started treatments with a massage therapist who used all manner of techniques—not to mention months of treatment with flower essences, the same alternative therapy my friend Bob used to treat his cancer, in which the distillation of flowers are thought to heal at the cellular level, beneficial to emotional healing since that is where memory is stored—to help cut my negative ties to the past. And it wasn't just Phil. It was a lifetime of everything from childhood abuse to abusive relationships to self-abuse, all of which belong in other stories. Tough job I'd given that massage therapist, and some people will laugh at me and call her efforts hocus pocus. But I'm here to tell you it works. I walked into her office in January 2011, looking for help with Phil's diabetes, a way to control his blood sugars without pharmaceuticals, not noticing that I was so sick with asthma I could barely breathe—I had become that used to it. I might not have engaged with her on a client basis had she not touched a few pressure points on my skull and stopped my wheezing and dried up my sinuses in about three seconds. Whether it was subconscious effort on my own behalf or there is actually something to her ancient craft, she converted me in that short period of time. I became a believer and submitted to ninety-minute sessions of deep-tissue massage, cranio-sacral release, Reiki, hypnosis, and guided imagery every three weeks, as well as daily dosing with the flower essences. Flower essences have also been used to great result ("Google" it!) to treat separation anxiety in pets. If only we had known, we still might have Tesla in our lives, too.

It all adds up to Phil and I moving together through a very dark time and then finding our way toward peace, even if occasionally I still have to remind him that I don't belong to anyone. But the birds and the squirrels finally moved back in: we even had a visit from the cedar waxwings this past spring. Phil and I, in general, reached the point of moving on from whatever vortex we were in, with food and the creation of meals as the thing we keep coming back to when relationship trials threaten to break up the ground we've gained.

Someday down the road, we'll rethink those wedding rings.

So there it is. A bona fide happy ending. We have learned, of course, what everyone must learn in life, and that is how to move beyond, which is actually what happy endings are. In the movies the hero and heroine land at ecstasy and glee and all is glowy and sweet, but what they never show is the dishes piling up, people farting, catching colds, waking up grumpy, gaining weight, losing weight, going bald, getting depressed, contracting disease. For us, however, we came to understand that food itself is medicine—and not just a way to get through it all. Am I grateful for the hardships? Maybe. Grateful is very closely related to grace, and I'd be a fool if I did not own up to the grace I'd been witness to these past few years. We learned. We overcame. And we grew. Simple as that.

We've all heard the saying, "That which does not kill you makes you stronger." Assuming you are also striving to keep your body healthy, it's true.

Or, as a wise colleague of mine once said: "A river is pulled just like the ocean by the moon. Think of the body as a river: restore its banks and let it follow its own direction, and the mind flows with it."

Acknowledgments

ALTHOUGH THIS IS A WORK OF NON-FICTION, names and certain identifying details have been altered. The information contained in this book is in no way meant to be prescriptive and is not meant to be a substitute for seeking medical care. It's simply the story of the way I've come to go about certain things. Never ingest any herb or food supplement without doing your own research first.

I'm grateful to my priceless editor, Julie Molinari, who saw this book much more clearly than I did, and Kate Burkett, who is perhaps the only human on the planet who could have ever gotten me to start Tweeting, Katherine Sears, Ken Shear, artist Kelsey Grafton, and all the production folks at Booktrope. It's a little bit amazing in our day and time to find a press that offers so much support and creative freedom to its authors. I also have to thank Nancy Casey, who nudged me forward and who said, "This story isn't finished yet." Proof positive that the one who sticks by you to the end is always the one you least expect.

Always and forever: Lance Olsen and Andi Olsen, for everything, just everything.

I also have to say thank you to my sons, G.H. and D.H., of whom I am so proud and who for over thirty years have been my compass, even when I'm sure to them it didn't seem like it.

And, it almost goes without saying: Deep gratitude, Pacman, for willingly serving as my anti-hero, because heroes are so boring.

Readers likely noticed that I've mentioned quite a few brand names along the way. No one has paid me to do this. I am a writer, not an ad agent. I mention exact names because those are the brands I used in creating the recipes, and I can attest to the quality of the recipes because I used certain products in them in a certain way. I can't guarantee outcomes where substitutions are used, but that's not to say experimentation isn't encouraged.

The following books and web addresses are places to go for more information on foods or nutritional data included in *Blue Moon Vegetarian*:

The New Laurel's Kitchen (2nd edition) by Laurel Robertson, Carol L. Flinders, and Brian Ruppenthal

Follow Your Heart's Vegetarian Soup Cookbook by Janice Cook Migliaccio

Moosewood Cookbook (1st edition) by Mollie Katzen

Conscious Cuisine by Chef Cary Neff

To Buy or Not to Buy Organic: What You Need to Know to Buy the Healthiest, Safest, Most Earth-Friendly Food by Cindy Burke

"My Friend the Garlic Scape" by Kim O'Donnel
http://blog.washingtonpost.com/mighty-appetite/2006/06/my_friend_the_garlic_scape_1.html

"Possible Link Between Vitamin D Deficiency, Alzheimer's Disease And Vascular Dementia" by Astrid Engelen
http://www.medicalnewstoday.com/articles/151458.php

"Great Plott! The toughest dog on the planet makes its debut at Westminster." by Richard B. Woodward
http://www.slate.com/articles/news_and_politics/heavy_petting/2008/02/great_plott.html

Oh She Glows' Our Perfect Veggie Burger Recipe
http://ohsheglows.com/2011/07/13/our-perfect-veggie-burger/

Lightlife
http://www.lightlife.com/

Natural Directions Organic
http://www.naturaldirections.com/

Butterfly Herbs, Inc.
http://www.butterflyherbs.com/

Tillamook Cheese
http://www.tillamookcheese.com/

Nancy's Cultured Dairy and Soy
http://www.nancysyogurt.com/

Don Pancho Authentic Mexican Foods
http://www.donpancho.com/

Umpqua Oats
http://www.umpquaoats.com/

Strictly Organic Coffee Company
http://www.strictlyorganic.com/

"Food-Related Illness and Death in the United States" by Paul S. Mead, Laurence Slutsker, Vance Dietz, Linda F. McCaig, Joseph S. Bresee, Craig Shapiro, Patricia M. Griffin, and Robert V. Tauxe of Centers for Disease Control and Prevention
http://wwwnc.cdc.gov/eid/article/5/5/99-0502.htm

ALSO BY PAULA MARIE COOMER

Summer of Government Cheese (Fiction - Short Stories) A collection of darkly introspective short stories. As they say, one way to dispel darkness is to expose it to light.

Dove Creek (General Fiction) After a disastrous and abusive marriage, single mother Patricia draws on her Cherokee roots for courage. She finds her place as a Public Health nurse, but she must constantly prove herself—to patients, coworkers, and family members—in her quest to improve the lives of others.

MORE GREAT READS FROM BOOKTROPE

Eat in Not Out-The Learn-How-to-Cook Book Without Recipes **by Melinda Hinson Neely** (How-to / Food & Nutrition) Learn to set up a kitchen, buy the right food, prepare simple and delicious meals, and eat healthy and economically with this helpful guide.

Discover more books and learn about our
new approach to publishing at **booktrope.com**.

Coomer, Paula Marie. author.
Blue moon vegetarian :
reflections, recipes, and
advice for a plant-based diet /

Made in the USA
San Bernardino, CA
02 December 2013